HYPERVENTILATION SYNDROME

BREATHING PATTERN DISORDERS
AND HOW TO OVERCOME THEM

Dinah Bradley

Illustrations by Sally Hollis-McLeod

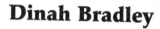

KYLE BOOKS

Dinah Bradley is a New Zealand trained and qualified physiotherapist with over 25 years' experience working in Britain, Australia and New Zealand. She has been involved in many areas of health care including childbirth education, geriatrics, neurology and respiratory medicine and has also worked as a freelance writer, photographer, TV researcher and a women's health activist.

Her published works include *Grandma's Teeth*, a picture book for children, *Becoming Single*, which she co-wrote with Hamish Keith, as well as editing the New Zealand edition of *Women's Health* by Sandra Cabot. Dinah Bradley is the co-author of *Multidisciplinary Approaches to Breathing Pattern Disorders* (Churchill Livingstone) as well as *Breathing Works for Asthma* with Tania Clifton-Smith, also for Kyle Books.

978 0 85783 029 6

A Cataloguing In Publication record for this title is available from the British Library.

Illustrations by Sally Hollis-McLeod
Printed and bound in Great Britain by Cox & Wyman Ltd, Reading, Berkshire

Contents

Foreword to the British Edition

It is with great pleasure that I write the foreword to a new edition of this excellent small book, which has been of great interest and practical use to many people (including many doctors and other health professionals) for a number of years. The need for an accurate and reliable source of information and instruction in this area is as great in 2011 as it was 20 years ago when the book first appeared.

It is probably true that there is a greater recognition of the various health problems that can be associated with abnormal breathing now than then, both amongst medical professionals and in the general public. Recent years have seen an expansion in scholarly articles and research in this field, with more rigorous scientific research underpinning the principles presented here. There is also more interest from the general media in the recognition and treatment of the overlapping problems of hyperventilation, dysfunctional breaching syndromes and breathing pattern disorders. However, there is little doubt that many people continue to suffer from avoidable illhealth and quality of life impairment because they are not breathing in a normal, healthy way.

The symptoms produced by abnormal breathing are characteristic but are not specific to breathing problems, and can cause difficulties in diagnosis and treatment. Doctors tend to be focussed on excluding important causes of breathlessness, chest discomfort and fatigue, and clearly it is vital that serious illnesses such as heart disease, asthma, anaemia and blood clots in the lung need to be found and treated. Unfortunately, when such illnesses are ruled out, other and more 'subtle' causes of symptoms are often forgotten about, and patients may come away thinking that they have been labelled as being neurotic or imagining their (very real!) symptoms, or that there is nothing that can be done to improve the situation. I am sure that there are many people all around the world in this situation, putting up with symptoms and curtailing their life and activities because of them. Even when suspected by the doctor or patient, there is often little availability of access to people who have expertise in treating such problems. This is a sad state of affairs, especially when the results of treatment by an appropriately skilled therapist can be so rewarding for the patient and the professional. Surveys indicate that as many as 1 in 10 people may have symptoms and quality of life impairment from abnormal breathing, and most won't have received a diagnosis or offered any treatment.

I hope that this situation is slowly improving! There is certainly more awareness now that many people with asthma can improve their symptoms from education and instruction in exercises designed to restore a more normal and 'functional' breathing pattern. However, there remains a real need for a concise and 'reader-friendly' book to explain how abnormal breathing can occur, what the effects of it are, and what can be done about it. In an ideal world, all with this problem would have access to a suitable skilled respiratory physiotherapist in a 'face to face' setting. Even then, it can be very helpful and reassuring to have a reliable source of information and instruction to refer to. For those finding it hard to understand their symptoms and to get help with them, such a book can be a lifeline.

Having had a clinical and research interest in this area for 20 years, one of the biggest problems that I have perceived is the lack of reliable information. We live in an 'information overload' era, and there are many people, seemingly knowledgeable and authoritative, claiming to understand the causes of ill health and offering ways of improving it. Unfortunately, in the field of breathing training, not all the information in the public arena bears up to close scrutiny, and sometimes misleading and exaggerated claims are made for different therapies. A simple, pragmatic and accessible source of accurate information and advice is therefore invaluable. This book has provided it for many years and continues to do so.

Dr. Mike Thomas PhD FRCP
Asthma UK Senior Research Fellow, University
of Aberdeen
Chief Medical Advisor, Asthma UK

Preface to the revised edition

My sister lent me an earlier edition of this book several years ago. I put it in my 'to read later' pile, and thought nothing more of it. A year later, two weeks before my 21st birthday – I landed in hospital as the result of a nasty chest infection, anaemia, the inevitable 'change of season', and my long-term asthma.

When I was first diagnosed with asthma and given the sticky, sugary Ventolin syrup, I was told I would grow out of it in my teens. My doctor also said 'breathe through your nose'. I tried. It was uncomfortable. I gave up. That was the only practical advice that anyone ever gave me, other than to 'take your medicine regularly'.

Until that major attack I had tried to ignore my asthma, although, looking back, there was no way I could. I was bound to it. I would feel powerless and panicky if I found myself somewhere without my puffer, and I had no reliable method to calm myself down. Graduating to steroid 'preventers' made it worse because now I had two inhalers to lug everywhere. And to use an inhaler in public felt like I was admitting to those around me that I was fit and unhealthy – even though I have always been a regular exerciser.

Although the hospital episode was a miserable and painful one, it was also the turning point in my attitude to my asthma. Interestingly, it wasn't being in hospital that panicked me. I was warm and well looked after, apart from the chain-smoking doctor who, without asking, trundled in with 10 medical students, tried to convince me that it was psychosomatic, and let me know that asthma gets worse for women in their early twenties.

The panic came when it was time to leave. Our house was being renovated, there was sawdust everywhere and that scared me. It was a windy day outside and that scared me. The idea of dancing at my own 21st scared me. The thought of setting foot inside a smoky bar terrified me, let alone getting to the end of a sentence in my broadcasting job. In short, in the hospital the medical staff and oxygen masks were in control of my lungs. Outside, it was just me.

After 21 years of letting other people (not) tell me what to do, and being a slave to my inhaler, I had developed a strong sense that there must be another way to gain power over my asthma. And since no one was offering, I had to ask around. At the asthma clinic where I'd been referred I asked if there was some sort of breathing specialist. That's when I met Dinah Bradley.

As we worked on my breathing technique, I remembered many things from the past: the doctor who said, 'Breathe through your nose,' acting classes where we had to 'breathe into our stomachs', the reason I got so tired during clothes-shopping expeditions ('hold your tummies in, girls!'). They were all things that make perfect sense but that I had to discover for myself because my experiences with the medical world were so, well, medicine-focused.

I cured my penchant for yawning, and learned how to breathe my way out of minor asthmatic irritations. I'm no longer scared to go anywhere or do anything, and if I'm caught somewhere without my inhaler, I can calm myself with my breathing, rather than let my breathing panic me (or I could just ask one-in-three New Zealand families for a puffer).

I consider other improvements in my life – sleeping well, regular exercise, no more depression, increased self-confidence and a generally happy disposition – to be a direct result of better breathing. It's the most fundamental of our human functions, and it's not until you can't take it for granted that you truly appreciate it. Best thing is, it's free.

Strangely, I only ever get panic attacks now when I see Dinah. I nervously check my breathing, make sure my posture is relaxed, and watch the imaginary bag of rice rise and fall. Why do I get nervous? Because she's one of the two women who changed my life. I'm the other one. It is so important to be your own health expert; I strongly urge you to take control of your own health, ask as many questions as you have to, explore every option available to you. And if someone gives you this book – read it'.

Gemma Gracewood
Television & Film Producer

Acknowledgements

Thanks and great appreciation to:

– Helen Benton and Bob Ross (Tandem Press NZ) for first publishing this book, in 1991. Further sincere thanks to Kyle Books for publishing this 20th anniversary edition.

– the late Dr. Claude Lum MA, MB, FRCP, FRACP for help and encouragement over the years, and for his illuminating writings on the subject.

– Dr. Mike Thomas for writing the foreword to this edition.

– my physiotherapy colleagues, especially the UK group Physiotherapy For Hyperventilation (www.physiohypervent.org).

– the increasing number for GPs and physicians and physiotherapists who now include breathing pattern disorders in their diagnostic repertoire.

Finally, to the many hundreds of patients who have offered such insight into this widespread and distressing disorder. Thank you.

Dinah Bradley
Respiratory Physiotherapist.
www.breathingworks.com

Introduction

In the twenty years since I wrote the first edition of this book, many, many people have written to tell me, or told me in person, how much they appreciate its message. It seemed to hit the right buttons for the huge group of people who suffered from this mysterious and then little-known stress disorder.

Hyperventilation syndrome – HVS – has been used as a descriptive title since the mid 1930s but it has been under intense scrutiny during the last decade. Some clinicians prefer the term breathing pattern disorders. In this edition I use both terms.

Learning about normal breathing patterns and balanced body chemistry is one aspect of recovery. Getting the chest muscles, neck and spine relaxed and working properly is another. Whether you can do this by yourself, or whether you need expert help, reading these accounts will help you sort out your priorities. Check with our website – www.breathing works.com for information and contacts.

Stress is essential to life. We'd be dead without it. But too much stress may also lead to our ending up dead. Leading the good life has been the human aim since the beginning of civilization, by achieving a balance between these two forces.

Energy efficient, physiologically balanced breathing is a vital part of this process.

PART 1

**All About
Hyperventilation
Syndrome/Breathing
Pattern Disorders**

One

What is Hyperventilation?

'You have to breathe to live. But if you breathe too much, life becomes dominated by fear of symptoms, and fear of living life to the full.'

Mike, 33

Hyperventilation means moving more air through the chest than the body can deal with. Most people have experienced hyperventilation – also called over-breathing – to some degree, usually in the form of an acute attack. It's a normal reaction to sudden danger or excitement, and the signs are easy to pick.

- Breathing and heart rates speed up.
- Adrenalin pours into the bloodstream.
- The nervous system is on 'red alert'.
- Muscles tense up.

Sometimes people faint or collapse – or find super-human reservoirs of strength. When the stressful event is over, the body returns to its normal relaxed state.

Less easy to spot is chronic hyperventilation, a

Hyperventilation Syndrome

breathing pattern disorder in which over-breathing becomes a habit – usually in response to prolonged stress or tension. More widespread symptoms are felt, and at times these appear out of the blue. The symptoms may mimic serious disease or remind the sufferer of the perhaps frightening events surrounding a past acute attack. When this happens more widespread symptoms mysteriously occur.

- Breathlessness at rest for no apparent reason
- Frequent deep sighs or yawning
- Chest-wall pains
- Palpitations
- Light-headedness and feeling 'spaced out'
- Tingling or numb lips or extremities
- Gut upsets or irritable bowel syndrome
- Achy muscles or joints, or tremors
- Tiredness, weakness, broken sleep, nightmares
- Sexual problems
- Clammy hands and high anxiety or phobias

Cascade of symptoms

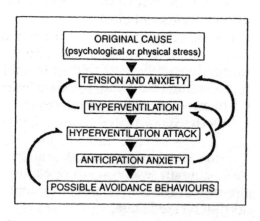

When over-breathing becomes chronic the balance between the oxygen-rich air we breathe in and carbon-dioxide-rich air we breathe out is upset: carbon dioxide levels start to drop.

Far from being just a waste gas at the end of the respiratory cycle, carbon dioxide is a powerful governor of many of the body's systems – including blood flow to the brain. With chronic over-breathing the normal acid/alkaline balance (pH) of the tissues is altered. The body becomes more alkaline, and the nerve cells are the first to respond to this respiratory alkalosis. Dizziness and tingling or numbness are often the first signs.

The autonomic nervous system, which looks after the body's involuntary functions (for example, heart rate, blood pressure and digestion), is affected too. This system is divided into two: the sympathetic, which governs action and 'get up and go', and the parasympathetic, which is responsible for rest, recuperation and calmness. Low carbon dioxide levels stimulate the sympathetic nervous system more than the parasympathetic, putting the body on continuous red alert.

If carbon dioxide levels in the blood fall further with continued over-breathing, body cells begin to produce lactic acid in an effort to balance their pH. Muscles ache. Metabolism is less efficient. Exhaustion and chronic tiredness soon follow, with feelings of physical and mental depression – all typical signs of long-term chronic hyperventilation.

Not only nerve cells are affected.

Muscle cells become more twitchy, and the smooth muscles of our blood vessels, airways and gut tighten and constrict in response to lowered carbon dioxide. There is an increased release of

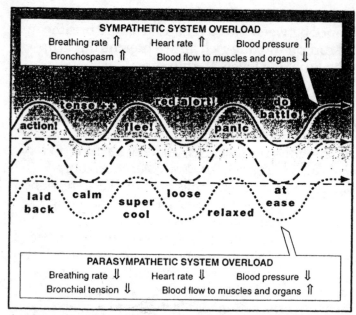

Autonomic nervous system, controller of involuntary body functions

histamines, which aggravates allergic responses. The heart starts pounding and the hyperventilator may feel panic-stricken, with palpitations and feelings of 'air hunger'.

When carbon dioxide levels are too low oxygen clings to its carriers – the red blood cells – and tissues, especially the brain, become starved of oxygen. The brain may have its oxygen supply cut by as much as 50 per cent, making it difficult to concentrate, let alone feel part of this planet. The drop in oxygen supply to the brain stimulates the breathing control centre to increase breathing rates and the chronic nature of the hyperventilation is reinforced.

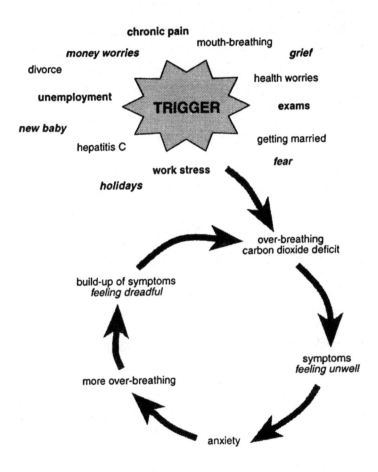

As the oxygen and carbon dioxide exchanges fuel every cell in our body, every system is ultimately going to be affected – leading to a distressing as well as puzzling range of symptoms.

Why does chronic hyperventilation happen?

Over-breathing is a normal reaction to stress or strain: it only becomes abnormal when stresses and strains reach levels that lead to chronic hyperventilation and outbreaks of symptoms. These stresses and strains may have *started* from:

• organic causes, for example, asthma, physical pain, pneumonia, anaemia, chronic chest or heart disease;
• physiological causes, for example, fever, high progesterone levels, prolonged talking, high altitude, diabetes, liver or kidney disease;
• psychological and social causes, for example, fear, anxiety, depression, perfectionist personality, separation/divorce, redundancy, unemployment, loneliness;
• drugs, for example, nicotine, caffeine, aspirin, amphetamines.

While these *original* causes may be dealt with, stabilised or cured, in certain people the respiratory centre in the brain is reset and the over-breathing becomes habitual. Even though the bad times are over, the increased breathing rate stays.

World-wide, the 1990s have been a decade of change and uncertainty. Our minds evolved in an ancestral environment that lacked the pressure, noise and speed of the present electronic age. We're constantly bombarded with information and our brains often can't cope with it all. We need to consciously take time out to counter this mega-stimulation, but few of us do.

The increase in stress disorders and diseases is alarming. Computerisation has pinned many workers in front of screens for extended periods of time, but the human body is not designed for prolonged sitting. We experience maximum stimulation from minimum effort and breathing is affected.

Adapting to rapid change is especially difficult if the change is unwanted or out of personal control. Stress levels soar, and with them adrenalin levels and heart rate, and nervous exhaustion follows – all fuelled by over-active lungs.

Is hyperventilation a modern disorder?

For centuries philosophers and scientists have understood the importance of good breathing. Hippocrates, the father of Western medicine, noted in the fifth century BC: 'The brain exercises the greatest power in mankind – but the air supplies sense to it.'

Adherents of both Buddhism, which originated in India also in the fifth century BC, and Taoism, from ancient China, combined breathing with relaxation and exercise to harmonise heart rate, breathing, digestion and circulation. Yoga and t'ai chi are modern versions of these ancient wisdoms.

Despite well-observed accounts in Western literature of 'breathless' heroines or heroes with their 'breath taken away', little was understood about the link between over-breathing and ill-health. The first detailed medical description of hyperventilation was not published until 1871, in a study of 300 American Civil War soldiers. A doctor noticed 'disabling shortness of breath, irritable heart and oppression of breathing' and thought the cause of these problems lay in the heart.

Around the turn of the century other medical researchers experimented with normal subjects, asking them to hyperventilate voluntarily; their results noted neurological effects (tingling and muscles spasms) as well.

The term hyperventilation syndrome (HVS) was coined in the 1930s. One British physician called it 'one of the commonest chronic afflictions of sedentary town dwellers'. Breathing into a paper bag (re-inhaling carbon dioxide-rich air) became a popular treatment for acute attacks of HVS at this time.

No theatre would be without a paper bag in the wings ready for stage-fright victims, frozen in respiratory alkalosis (terror) while awaiting their cue. However, while the paper bag method may be useful in helping with acute panic attacks, it is of no use to chronic over-breathers. It may temporarily restore normal blood gases, but it does nothing to correct the underlying cause – breathing pattern disorders.

It is extremely dangerous during an acute asthma attack to try to control rapid wheezy breathing using a paper bag. Increased drives to breathe are normal during an attack. It is on record that at least one person has breathed their last into a brown paper bag.

Recent medical research has revealed more about the physiological system derangements, metabolic imbalances and anxiety-related symptoms caused by habitual over-breathing, but it is still an under-recognised and under-treated disorder.

Whether it is primarily a mental or a physical health problem has been hotly debated. Fortunately, the move towards holistic medicine, in which body and soul are treated together, has been of benefit to the vast number of people suffering from chronic hyperventilation and to their doctors, who can add this distressing disorder to their diagnostic repertoire.

'I had a medical file as thick as a phone book and I always seemed to be at the doctors having tests for this and that. Nothing was ever found to be really wrong. But a locum picked it straight away. My breathing was grossly askew and my symptoms were a result of this. At last I had something to work on.'

Joan, 54

Who Develops Breathing Pattern Disorders?

'When I went to the physiotherapist for breathing retraining, my daughter took me with her nine-year-old son – my grandson – who was off school. It was really funny seeing how we all breathed alike, and had little habits the same. We all had disordered patterns – all three generations.'

Ann, 63

All sorts of people develop breathing pattern disorders, and at all ages.

• Children are not exempt. Chronic blocked noses and habitual mouth-breathing often establish chaotic breathing patterns from quite early ages.
• People with asthma – about 15 per cent of New Zealand's population – are particularly prone to chronic hyperventilation. With recent advances in user-friendly inhalers to manage symptoms, few benefit from breathing retraining and physical therapies to improve respiratory function and the mechanical changes to the neck and chest muscles common in over- breathers.
• Following major surgery, some people find the

breathing techniques encouraged at the time of their operation – very big in-breaths to re-expand the lungs after anaesthesia – trigger hyperventilation during recovery. With the rapid turn-around in hospitals, or by having to travel to other centres for treatment, some do not receive post-operative care to correct this problem. (It's best to concentrate on restoring low, slow nose/abdominal breathing and relaxation in between bouts of 'big breathing' and coughing.)

• Those with more permanent lung damage – chronic obstructive airway diseases or emphysema, for instance – often develop inefficient breathing patterns, with HVS adding to their stress levels.

• People with heart disease and hypertension may also find that anxiety about health adds to their HVS symptoms. While medication to manage the disease is prescribed, often little attention is paid to the co-existing breathing disorder.

• Some women are extra sensitive to hormonal changes, either in the week before their period or in the second half of pregnancy. Higher progesterone levels increase respiratory drives. Carbon dioxide levels may be reduced by up to 25 per cent, inducing HVS symptoms.

• Menopause, with its hormonal fluctuations, is also a common cause of breathing pattern disorders.

• Older people facing retirement or redundancy may have problems adjusting to ageing, loss or erratic health. They are prime candidates for breathing pattern disorders.

• HVS is surprisingly common amongst teenagers with raging hormones, peer pressures, parental expectations and educational and recreational demands adding up to 'major mega-stress'.

• Victims of abuse or torture often suffer chronic breathing pattern disorders and sympathetic system overload, with a frightening array of symptoms adding to their distress.
• Migrant groups, adjusting to a new culture while grieving for their own, frequently have breathing-related disorders, especially if they are from earthquake, flood or war zones.
• High achievers and workaholics who put huge pressures on themselves are sitting ducks for HVS. High stress levels equate with sympathetic system overload.

No one is immune, as the following accounts show.

Jane, 36

My first attack of acute hyperventilation happened at a street parade. It was hot, crowded and noisy, and I left my husband and two kids to find some shade.

I couldn't stay still and paced up and down feeling terrible. Then my hearing went and I felt dizzy, as though I might faint. But I didn't and nothing seemed to change for about 15 minutes or so. I could see a policeman nearby so I felt fairly safe.

I found my husband and got the keys to go back to the car. He could see I wasn't well so we went home. I went to my doctor the next morning. He took about 20 tubes of blood and tested for everything – and they all came back negative. His diagnosis was that I had a virus – even though all the tests said I was in good health. I spent two weeks in bed, but after three weeks I still felt terrible so I abandoned the virus idea. I then went to another doctor for a second opinion and he diagnosed an anxiety disorder.

He said it would go away, and no other help was offered. I didn't really know what to think about that diagnosis. I certainly *was* anxious about my symptoms, and I dreaded attacks.

I got heaps of self-help books – I had them stacked up by my bed. But I only looked at them: I couldn't actually do anything. I wasn't sleeping much by then either. By now I was convinced I had a huge brain tumour that the doctors weren't telling me about. How could I continue to feel so spaced out and ill, yet all my tests be OK?

One evening not long after this I insisted on going to an accident and emergency clinic: I was about to die. There were around 20 people waiting, and I looked at all these sick people ahead of me. I couldn't wait for them. After all, they were only sick – I was dying! We raced into the pharmacy next door to ask the chemist to help me (like the ad on television says to do). He peered over his glasses and pigeon-holed me instantly as a 'flake'. He didn't think I was dying.

'I bet your house is tidy,' he said. 'You can come down and dust this place any time.' He thought I was a rather extreme example of the 'worried well' with a dash of over-achiever's zeal.

I begged for something to take to help me at least sleep. He suggested a strong over-the-counter sedative which would make me feel awful (he wasn't going to let me off lightly) but I would sleep, and said that if it didn't work my husband should give me a good clip round the ear. It was all very jokey, but no help at all to me or my husband.

I was getting frantic by now. Every scan, test and

x-ray showed I was well, but I still had symptoms. The dizzies, achy muscles (especially my upper chest, neck and shoulders), terrible gut upsets. I felt so unwell I had to give up my part-time job – a job I really loved. I didn't even want to go out.

I heard about HVS and went to a respiratory physiotherapist to have that checked out. I hadn't been aware of my breathing except for the feeling I wasn't getting enough air – which I interpreted on an emotional level (*I was going to die*) – and sighing all the time, and hunching my shoulders up.

The lengthy assessment showed my breathing rates and patterns were all over the shop, and, mechanically, that my upper chest was doing all the work and I was holding myself tight round my waist – through all the anxiety and fear. I was mouth-breathing all the time too. It felt really uncomfortable when I tried to nose-breathe. I was pushing truckloads more air through my chest than normal.

Going back over my history it became apparent that the attack I had at the parade was a severe acute attack on top of what was probably long-standing chronic over-breathing. So what seemed like normal after my dreadful episode was over wasn't normal at all. In fact my resting breathing rate was 24 a minute. (Normal is half that.)

We found, too, that things had been building up over many years, unnoticed or attributed to something else. My symptoms were worse premenstrually, and when I thought back to my pregnancies I realised I probably had had undiagnosed post-natal depressions. Not long before the parade disaster I'd been obliged to work full-time for a couple of months to cover for someone else – of course I couldn't say no. And that had been one of the last straws on the camel's back. For a long time I'd been running on empty but kept on going – just like everyone else. Hell, I was young and healthy.

Because I'd been in this spiral for so long I was in such a mess that I agreed to have some counselling as well, and to go on anti-anxiety pills. These particular ones are good at muscle relaxation and stopping me being on 'red alert' all the time. I was very reluctant to take pills, but when I understood that the drug replaced stuff I wasn't producing enough of – serotonin – because of my stress, and that I needn't stay on them forever, I agreed. I hated it at first, but I stuck it out and after about six weeks it knocked the top off most of my anxieties.

It's given me space to work on the physical stuff – breathing properly again. Getting my physiology right and learning to relax, to let go – that's been unbelievably hard. Back to the beginning really, as my physio said. Just as it took me a long time to become unwell, it'll take time to become well. I have to be patient – and do the work.

Tom, 6
as told by his mother

The school nurse rang to say Tom was in the infirmary with stomach pains, and asked if I would come and pick him up. Even though he was the picture of health, he had been complaining of sore stomachs prior to this as well as other vague symptoms. He was happy at school and doing well. I thought he was breathing strangely though (I'd read about breathing pattern disorders in a magazine so I was alert to a possible problem). He seemed to hunch his shoulders up and take big breaths into his upper chest through his mouth. I took him to our doctor for a check-up. She couldn't find anything wrong. I asked for a referral for physiotherapy, which she reluctantly agreed to. I think she thought I was being too fussy.

During our first session Tom was asked all sorts of questions, and what came out was truly bizarre. During physical education Tom's teacher had told the boys that girls breathed with their stomachs and boys breathed with their upper chests. The manly look was to puff out your upper chest. He apparently singled Tom out as an example of 'girl' breathing. The poor boy! He'd been struggling to be an upper-chest breather, but not only did it not feel right, it made him feel sick. He was so pleased to know 'tummy breathing' was normal.

He had no problems getting back to 'normal' breathing. And the physio had an interesting conversation with his teacher!

Dan, 51

The first symptoms appeared in June last year. I was sailing with my wife and there'd been storm warnings and the worries that go with that. (We were living on our boat.) One may assume that anxiety and apprehension were the cause of what happened next: erratic breathing, pain in the top of my head, and an overall feeling of exhaustion which lasted about an hour. My recovery was speedy once we got safely underway.

The next incident was in December, also on the boat, but in ideal conditions and a non-stressful environment – a sudden feeling of dizziness, a pain in the head and I semi-fainted. As quick as it happened, I recovered. But a couple of hours later, getting out of the dinghy, my knees went wobbly and I had to slump back until I recovered a few minutes later. A doctor's appointment was made as a result of these frightening incidents, but after all sorts of tests nothing could be detected that may have caused the attacks. I was advised to take aspirin daily – the doctor thought blood-clotting in the neck area may have been a factor.

In January I had further attacks, which my wife put down to nerves as there were some atrocious sailing conditions. Always afterwards there was the feeling of exhaustion.

Back home, my doctor thought I might have been having hyperventilation problems and booked me in for assessment with a breathing specialist.

Two days before my appointment, on the second day of a new job, I experienced another attack of breathlessness, dizziness and disorientation. My whole body felt as though I was in an earthquake, but no one else could see this. I was driven to the hospital; following extensive tests, including several blood tests, it was revealed my carbon dioxide levels were very, very low. When I had my appointment with the physio, a breathing disorder was confirmed.

As a result of two visits, I have an awareness of the problem and the ability to deal with it. The problem has hardly arisen, and if it does it can be countered easily.

For what it's worth, over the years I'd had a broken marriage, remarriage, problems with teenagers from two families that greatly affected me, early retirement from the police force from burn-out – all these were contributing factors. But what was so puzzling was that it was not until all these stresses were behind me and we were enjoying our new lifestyle that the symptoms appeared.

Fortunately it was treated quickly.

Kate, 24

I'd been feeling a bit run-down, but I couldn't take a break. I'd just started my first job as a lawyer in a big law firm and I put in a lot of extra time. Missed meals and late nights – I had a fairly active social life as well – took their toll.

I started feeling breathless running up stairs, and I found the gym much harder than usual. People noticed I was sighing a lot too – not a good look with clients.

I had other odd symptoms as well, like feeling light-headed, so I checked up with my GP. I was anaemic – I had a low red blood cell count. My doctor pointed out the red blood cells were the ones that carry the oxygen round the body. That's why I'd been feeling breathless – not enough oxygen carriers.

That was successfully treated, and I thought that'd be it – but I still had funny symptoms. It was an ambulance officer who told me I was hyperventilating, at a football match of all places. I checked on the internet and found hundreds of references on the subject. It seems to be a widespread and common disorder. And even though I was no longer anaemic, I was still over-breathing from habit. This was treated by physiotherapy; I was only too keen to work on retraining my breathing back to normal. I'm symptom-free now.

Mary, 30

I was 24, recently married and newly pregnant with my first baby. We had moved from one city to another and I really missed my family. I had a successful business – four florist shops, which meant a lot of early morning starts at the flower market and staff organisation. There was a lot of pressure which I managed well at first.

I worked right up until the day before my daughter was born, and it was a difficult birth. I was back at work four days later. The first business meeting I had to go to after this was when I had my first attack. I felt panic-stricken and I went bright red, sweating and shaking. I had to leave the meeting. My fingers curled up and went stiff – it was terrifying.

My husband rushed me to the doctor. My blood pressure was up and my heart was racing. Because of concern about my blood pressure, my doctor sent me to be checked by a specialist physician. One thing's worse than high blood pressure, and that's worrying about it. I was very distressed.

The specialist shook my hand when we met and listened to my story.

He said he knew exactly what was wrong with me just by shaking my hand (very clammy!). He also pointed out – my husband had noticed too – that my breathing was fast and full of big sighs. He gave me a complete medical examination, more to put my mind at rest than anything else. Every test was normal. I felt very at ease and I trusted this man, but deep down I just couldn't believe that there wasn't something wrong with me. I was in a very bad way.

He sent me for physiotherapy to improve my breathing, as well as counselling, but I had no one to help me get there – I hadn't built up a network of friends to help with my baby, or me. I was desperate to get there, but I missed appointments. I felt even more unwell, and helpless.

I did eventually get to a couple of appointments but I still couldn't believe there wasn't something really wrong. I went back to the physician and he sent me off for a brain scan, just to reassure me. Over the next five years I had six brain scans – can you believe it – all normal, of course. Plus every other test you can think of. I estimate trying to find a diagnosis cost over $10,000.

I've had five years of slipping and sliding, but with counselling and regular physiotherapy checks I've taken responsibility for my own wellness. I've made lifestyle changes to reduce stress. I take time for relaxation and time for exercise, and I no longer feel guilty about taking that time. I know my danger signs. I know what to do and why – and it works.

Jack, 62

I had a mild heart attack about 10 years ago, which gave me a fright. It made me give up smoking. I made a good recovery and was pretty well until a couple of years ago, when I started getting angina. Tests showed I had coronary artery disease and I was scheduled for heart surgery for a triple bypass. It was very successful and, although I had a few breathing difficulties after the operation, I was up and about quickly and felt tremendous benefit. The exercises I had to do after the op were designed to expand the lungs to prevent chest infections. I had this little gadget to encourage me to breathe in deeply. I got into the habit then of breathing in hard and using my upper chest.

Anyway, a few months down the track I had sharp upper chest pains which worried me. But when I went for a check-up, my heart was fine. The cardiologist then sent me to a respiratory physician to check my lungs. They were OK too, but the way I was breathing was not. They diagnosed hyperventilation. My breathing rate was 26 a minute, and I was a mouth breather. My wife had noticed this as well. When I put my hand on my breastbone I could feel my upper chest working like bellows.

The chest doctor sent me for physiotherapy, which I must say has been extremely helpful, not only helping me get back to normal energy-efficient breathing, but also sorting out the aches and pains in my chest and shoulders. I'm sleeping well again, and garden and exercise with confidence.

3

What Is 'Good Breathing'?

'My son reckons I'm contributing to global warming, the way I've been breathing. He's always on at me about increased carbon dioxide emissions!'

Rob, 44

'Good breathing' means moving air in and out of the chest with the minimum of effort and using the chest muscles to their best advantage.

Three main groups of muscles are used for breathing.

The diaphragm

Tailor made for each person to supply the right amount of air to the lungs during rest and normal activity, this strong, thin, flat sheet of muscle is attached to the lower edges of the ribs. It separates the chest from the gut.

Shaped rather like the dome of an umbrella, it flattens down to expand the lungs. That's why your stomach expands as you breathe in. It draws in oxygen-rich air with very little effort. As the diaphragm relaxes the dome shape is restored and carbon dioxide-rich air is gently exhaled. Diaphragmatic movement can vary from 1 centimetre at rest to 10 centimetres during exercise.

It acts as a vital pump helping the heart to circulate blood up and down the body, and its gentle action on the stomach helps digestion as well as lymphatic flow.

Diaphragmatic or abdominal breathing is the most energy- efficient and relaxed way to breathe and it helps reduce sympathetic tone (see page 20).

Chest or intercostal muscles

These muscles join the ribs together and tighten to lift them, like a bird's wings, expanding the chest walls to draw in air and contracting back to push air out (see page 40).

They use about 20 per cent more energy than the diaphragm.

In quiet breathing the lower ribs flare gently, helping the diaphragm, while the upper ribs remain relaxed. During moderate to strong exercise the upper chest opens up, like a reserve tank, to draw in extra oxygen-rich air; this also happens in response to fear or anger.

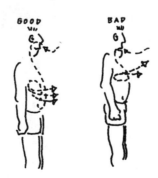

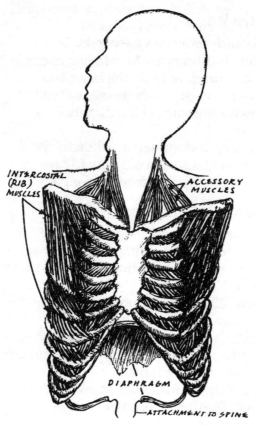

INTERCOSTAL
(RIB)
MUSCLES

ACCESSORY
MUSCLES

DIAPHRAGM

ATTACHMENT TO SPINE

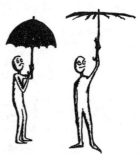

Accessory muscles

The neck and shoulder muscles are used to tense and lift the upper chest in order to increase upper chest volumes; you can feel them working after strenuous exercise or effort. They work all the time in adults with breathing rates of 20 or more a minute.

Stomach muscles are accessory muscles too, and you can feel those helping with breathing out during moderate to heavy exercise.

In normal, relaxed breathing 70-80 per cent of the work is done by the diaphragm, and the lower chest muscles do about 20–30 per cent. The accessory muscles are on stand-by for extremes of effort or stress. Habitual hyperventilators tend to reverse this ratio.

Oxygen and carbon dioxide levels, or blood gases, are kept in healthy balance by 12 regular breaths a minute (10–14 breaths is the normal range for adults). This moves 3–5 litres of air through the chest each minute.

Chronic over-breathers exchange up to double this amount of air. They are able to increase

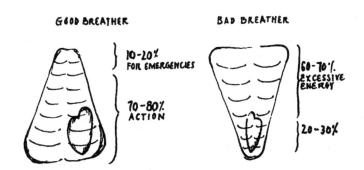

GOOD BREATHER   BAD BREATHER

10-20% FOR EMERGENCIES

70-80% ACTION

60-70% EXCESSIVE ENERGY

20-30%

volumes by switching from nose- to mouth-breathing. The next section explains why nose-breathing is important to respiratory health and the restoration of a normal energy-efficient breathing pattern.

Winning by a nose

'When I came to after surgery to my nose – injured playing football – I was in a blind panic. Both nostrils were packed with dressings and I felt I was suffocating. Breathing through my mouth felt so out of control and was making me feel very strange. My hands and lips were tingling. I rang the bell for help and the nurse was pretty abrupt with me. She said, "You're just hyperventilating," and virtually told me to get a grip and calm down. Boy, if she'd felt like I felt, she might have been a bit more helpful. Unfortunately that experience stuck with me and I had a lot of trouble with my breathing for a few months. I was as crook as a dog some days. Fortunately my GP was on to it and sent me off to physio for some breathing retraining. I only needed one check-up after the first session and it was quite an education. My breathing's good now.'
Jeff, 25

One of the commonest findings in patients with breathing pattern disorders is chronic mouth-breathing. Many have untreated nasal or sinus problems. The nose and nasal health have been woefully neglected in general medicine in recent times. Unless the person is sent to an ear, nose and throat specialist for serious nasal problems, not much attention seems to be paid to the less dramatic but disturbing effects of chronic nasal airflow problems – by either sufferer or doctor.

I talked to a paediatrician recently who honestly admitted that, as long as his asthmatic patients slept through the night and could go to school, he didn't bother much about their nasal stuffiness and resulting mouth-breathing patterns.

How the nose works

Our sense of smell is very important. It rests in the rhinencephalon, an area of the brain that developed early in our evolution and still has primitive connections to many other body systems that are vital to our survival. While our noses have lost some of their finer 'sniffing' abilities, they still have a vital role in guarding our respiratory health.

Watch a dog trotting round the neighbourhood sniffing all the various 'news stands' on the way, gathering vast amounts of information about friends and foes. We probably get as much information reading the daily newspaper.

The sense of smell is important to our emotional health too – smell can trigger memories of good and bad environments, good and bad people, sad or happy times. It has links with many – other vital body functions, such as the heart, the lungs and the gut – through intriguing and complex reflexes and nerve connections.

The most obvious nasal reflex is the sneeze. The nasal linings co-ordinate with many other reflexes from the brain and spinal cord to produce a spontaneous 'aa-choo' to clear irritants from the upper airways.

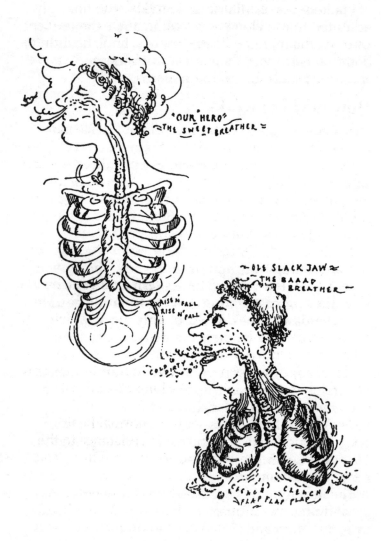

Body temperature is influenced by the temperature of the air breathed out of the nose. And think how powerful our nasal reflexes are in response to fumes. Very strong irritants can reduce or even stop breathing temporarily, and affect the heart rate. Milder stimulants cause a reflex increase in breathing. This is why some people feel bad in shopping malls or aeroplanes: their symptoms are triggered by over-breathing in response to air fresheners or the 'scents of the day' pumped into the air-conditioning systems.

Breathing through the nostrils draws air over fine filtering hairs into the inner nose – then through turbinates, baffles and nasal linings, swirling the air around so it is warmed and humidified in preparation for the lung.

Air breathed in through the mouth misses out on this 'air-conditioning'.

The nose not only has two external nostrils, but two inner noses, divided by the nasal septum, that work together. One dilates to carry the major part of the air stream while the other rests, or clears out any debris. During waking hours these rhythmic cyclic changes happen every two to four hours. You can check this yourself by blocking one nostril to see which side is on duty.

Breathing through the nose, in normal health, there is roughly 50 per cent more resistance to the air flow in contrast to mouthbreathing. This becomes obvious when you switch from nose- to mouth-breathing – try it yourself. This resistance creates pressure differences between the external nose and the lung, which are essential for efficient respiration.

It's interesting that this lowering of resistance

was what Jeff found so distressing when he was forced to mouth-breathe after his nasal surgery. Fortunately, very few surgeons pack nostrils post-operatively.

Sleep and nasal congestion

If you sleep on your side, the lower nostril tends to congest while the upper nostril takes over. The head – and body – turn to reverse this pattern; these turning cycles are part of restful healthy sleep. The cycling rates vary with sleep patterns.

Sleeping in one position can lead to cramps, neck stiffness, back ache, erratic breathing and poor rest. Having too many turning cycles – thrashing about – is also unrestful. This is often caused by poor nasal and respiratory function during sleep, as anyone who has recently had a head cold will confirm.

Chronic snoring with interrupted breathing during sleep combined with daytime sleepiness needs further investigation. If you have this problem you should discuss it with your doctor.

Long sequences of nights spent in unrefreshing sleep lead to a multitude of problems. Tension and anxiety, vivid dreams or nightmares, poor concentration, chronically disturbed breathing patterns; all these become part of feeling generally 'stressed out'.

Sleeping with the mouth closed can be hard. When you're really relaxed the jaw relaxes too, with the mouth falling open. There's not much you can do about that short of wearing a chin-strap like Monsieur Poirot, or taping your lips together as recommended by Buteyko practitioners. At least try going off to sleep breathing through your nose. Don't worry if you wake with a dry mouth – as long as you slept well and wake refreshed.

Breathe Right™ nasal strips, which stick to the outside of the nostrils, dilating them, can be of great benefit in getting used to nose-breathing at night.

Medical treatments

When the nose becomes congested the nasal sinuses (hollow areas in the supporting facial bones) become prime sites for inflammation and infection. Allergic reactions to inhaled irritants cause rhinitis or hayfever in susceptible people, also a trigger for chronic sinusitis; post nasal drip puts the lower airways and lungs at risk of infection. Mixtures of allergic reactions and chronic infections are common and can be very tricky to treat.

Nose-blowing, if too violent, can also cause sinus and ear problems. The best way to blow your nose and prevent damage to the tubes that connect with the inner ear is to block off one nostril while clearing the other *gently*. Teach your children by example.

Sorting out nasal and sinus problems takes a lot of detective work and patience. It's worth starting with a nasal scan if the problems are chronic. Only slightly more expensive than an x-ray, a nasal scan shows far more accurately the state of the nose and sinuses. You and your doctor can then be more specific with treatment options rather than the hit and miss approach of trying (and wasting) different sprays or drops – in the blind hope they'll work.

If your doctor prescribes a nasal medication, make sure you know exactly what it's for, why you're taking it and how to use it, and ask about and be prepared for any side-effects. It is worth putting up with short-term discomfort for long-term relief.

Nasal medications fall into two groups.

• Relievers in the short term cause shrinkage of the nasal linings. They can be used intermittently, but mustn't be used continuously because overuse makes the nose clog up even more.
• Preventers have long-term anti-inflammatory and anti-allergic benefits. These are usually local steroids which coat the lining of the nose with minimal effect on the rest of the body. Commitment to regular use for long periods is essential to get the full benefit.

Both relievers and preventers come in drops, sprays and aerosols. Sometimes it helps to have a change if one method seems ineffective.

Over-the-counter pills from chemists are useful for seasonal allergies. Antibiotics may be prescribed by your doctor to knock out bacterial infection (the full course must be taken).

Physiotherapy offers ultrasound electrotherapy, pressure point treatments and acupuncture (worth a try if you're anti-drugs).

Alternative remedies

There are also some old, inexpensive treatments that can be very effective in the early stages of infection.

Try steam inhalations with eucalyptus oil or

Friars Balsam. Talk to your chemist – some stock inhalation pots with shaped tops to direct the steam; these are safer to use than open bowls for younger children, the very elderly or those with disabilities. Wear a shower cap to protect your hair.

Nasal rinse

We recommend using the sinus rinse sachets available from all chemists. But if you want to make your own solution, here is the recipe. Clean a 1200ml glass bottle carefully, then fill it with bottled water. (You need not boil this water.) Use 2–3 heaped teaspoons of rock salt. Do not use table salt as it contains additives. Add 1 rounded teaspoon of baking soda (pure bicarbonate). Store at room temperature and shake or stir before each use. Mix a new batch weekly. Boil water for 3 minutes if using tap water. An easy way to prepare the solution is to purchase a glass bottle of still water and continue as above – this will last you all week, and you can re-use the bottle.

Check out the health shop: there are many naturopathic remedies that may work for you. They can be expensive, so ask for supporting literature.

Exercise is another treatment alternative – heel strike in running or brisk walking helps vibrate the sinus cavities. The nasal airways dilate and circulation increases with aerobic exercise, helping sinus drainage.

Think about some external causes of nasal problems and how you can fix, change or avoid them:

• allergies (no more cats sleeping on the bed, for instance)

- environmental pollution (smoky pubs, dusty or dirty workplaces)
- mechanical obstruction (polyps or injury).

Think about the internal causes too.

With chronic breathing pattern disorders, the breathing control centre in your brain is keen to keep you over-breathing, and the mouth is the easiest route. Unfortunately air is not warmed, filtered or humidified when you mouth-breathe; the nose is a built-in air-conditioner.

Relearning nose-breathing can be very uncomfortable at first. Those who can't get the knack need to get help – book in with a respiratory physiotherapist. Be kind to your lungs.

Nasal health is a top priority in restoring normal breathing patterns and better health – in the most surprising areas.

'The most radical part of learning to nose-breathe again was I could kiss properly. My boyfriend pointed out to me that kissing me used to be like kissing a gasping goldfish. And it's made the rest of my sex life so much better too, because I feel so much better. I hadn't realised what I was missing out on.'

Emma, 26

4

Why Do People Become Hyperventilators?

'Someone recently pointed out that how many
hours a week you work has almost become a
status symbol. I and most of my contemporaries
put in a 60-hour week and I admit we do tend to
boast about it. But the pressure I put myself under
– it's killing.'
Dave, 37

The respiratory centre in the hind-brain responds to
messages from different parts of the body, as well
as from the higher brain or cerebral cortex. After a
bout of rapid breathing, whether from hard
exercise, high emotions or danger, the respiratory
system gradually allows the breathing rate to slow
down as the body regains balanced blood gases.

In those under *prolonged* stress, the respiratory
centre adapts gradually to accept lower or
fluctuating carbon dioxide levels and respiratory
alkalosis. Various parts of the body and mind may
feel extremely uncomfortable with the blood gas
imbalances, but the respiratory centre rides
roughshod over any distress signals it receives: it
keeps instructing the lungs to breathe hard and fast.

The causes for this may be mechanical, starting

after chest surgery or in lung diseases which cause airflow disturbances, for example, bronchiectasis and tuberculosis. The disorder may start after physical illnesses such as pneumonia, chest infections, glandular fever and viral infections.

HVS often appears during or after emotional upheavals:

- death of a spouse, lover or relative
- separation or divorce
- losing a job
- changes of status; growing up; ageing
- moving to a different town
- living in a war zone.

Exercise, too, may trigger hyperventilation attacks when stress levels are high and fitness levels are low.

What does it feel like to hyperventilate?

The most common phrases hyperventilators use are:

- 'I thought I was going to pass out – I couldn't seem to take the next breath in.'
- 'I never seem to get a satisfying breath.'
- 'I've never been quite the same since my operation.' (Or accident, or break-up . . .)
- 'I really thought I was losing my mind.'
- 'I thought I was dying.'

In sudden attacks people are usually less aware of heaving upper-chest breathing but are all too aware of the anxiety and strange symptoms that might follow, such as dizziness, tingling fingers and lips, and panicky thoughts.

Those who rush to their doctor may be prescribed a mild tranquilliser after a full check-up and reassurance that 'nothing's wrong'. For some this is enough to break the cycle. But others who find their strange and frightening symptoms recur are left to imagine the worst:

> **Heart attack!**
> **Brain tumour!**
> **Bowel cancer!**

Do they go back to their doctor, or write their will?

Once the breathing pattern becomes centred in the upper chest and away from the diaphragm, more widespread and frightening symptoms begin to emerge, and a 'Catch 22' cycle is established.

Is hyperventilation syndrome very common?

The short answer is yes.

One group of European researchers described HVS as a 'silent epidemic'. British figures suggest that up to 40 per cent of patients sitting in GPs' waiting rooms have disordered breathing patterns. Specialists attract high numbers too, with an estimated 50–70 per cent of patients habitually over-breathing.

No New Zealand-wide studies have been published on the prevalence of HVS in specialist or general practice, but various studies from emergency coronary care unit admissions for acute chest pain have revealed that 30–40 per cent of suspected heart attack victims had absolutely nothing wrong with their hearts.

No figures are available from alternative health care sources.

The hazards of heavy breathing

• Habitual mouth-breathers develop irritable upper airways, with the risk of repeated upper respiratory tract infections. A very common sign of hyperventilation is repeated throat clearing: the a-hrrrrrm bug.

• Chronic over-breathing triggers increased histamine levels in the blood. Sweaty palms and flushed cheeks are signs of this. Those with allergies – and this includes people with asthma, hayfever, food intolerances and skin rashes – find their symptoms get worse.

• Response to pain is amplified, with stiffness, aching and tension in muscles, tendons and joints resulting from chronic hyperventilating and poor metabolism.

• Heart-disease-type symptoms, such as chest-wall tightness or pain and palpitations, can be downright terrifying.

• Mental fuzziness, headaches or memory lapses erode self-confidence, especially if work suffers.

• Making love can become a nightmare – for both partners – if the heavy breathing needed to reach orgasm leads to a panic attack.

• Vivid or bad dreams and disturbed sleep patterns often accompany hyperventilation, making for round-the-clock distress and exhaustion.

Almost every system in the body suffers. Fear of the relentless symptoms drives the respiratory centre into top gear and the cycle is complete. Hyperventilation syndrome gives free rein to the

fear . . . and the symptoms . . . and the
bewilderment of the sufferer, family and friends.

'It was a mystery to me how Susie, once so
outgoing and full of energy, had turned into a
fearful, tired shadow of her old self. I admit I
wasn't very sympathetic. It was tough on our kids.
I had no idea what to do or who to turn to.'

Edward, 40

5

What Can I Do about HVS?

'Within two months I'd been to the emergency department six times with chest pains and breathing very fast. I had pins and needles and felt sick each time. I had lots of different tests and nothing was wrong. This last time a doctor I hadn't seen before immediately diagnosed hyperventilation and sent me off for physiotherapy treatment.'

Mele, 42

As yet there is no reliable repeatable laboratory test to confirm a diagnosis of HVS, but after a thorough check-up to rule out organic disease your doctor may check for HVS in several ways.

The doctor may use skilled observation to detect irregular or fast breathing patterns, or signs of sympathetic system overload (rapid pulse, sweating, jumpiness).

You may do the 'think test', in which breathing patterns are monitored as you talk about symptoms and anxieties. Most people can pinpoint a stressful event which, when brought to mind, triggers most of their symptoms, along with increased breathing rates or sighs.

You might be asked to take the 12-breath test, an exercise in voluntary over-breathing. To many sufferers' amazement this can reproduce exactly their distressing symptoms. It is more useful as a teaching tool than as an accurate diagnostic test.

There are three main types of chest pain associated with hyperventilation syndrome.

• Sharp pains felt breathing in, often just below the left breast, from pressure on the diaphragm from a bloated stomach, filled by 'air-gulping', causing spasm of the diaphragm and pain.
• Dull aching chest-wall soreness, often felt after exercise; this is due to overstretching of chest-wall (intercostal) and accessory muscles, or from the heart itself banging on the inside of the chest wall.
• Heavy pain behind the breast-bone radiating to the neck and arms; this happens when the blood supply to the heart muscle itself is reduced in response to altered blood chemistry from chronic over-breathing with spasming of the coronary arteries.

Unfortunately all three types of pain are difficult to reproduce on demand: the multiple stressors (physical, social, emotional) that combine with hyperventilating to bring on chest pain are not found in the security of your doctor's rooms.

Other more high-tech methods of diagnosis are available but because blood gas levels fluctuate in chronic hyperventilators it may be difficult to pick up the problem from a single test. More often than not, it's a matter of ruling out what it *isn't*.

Unfortunately, for your doctor to test you for

hyperventilation he or she needs to be aware of the disabling effect of the condition. It may be reassuring to be told, 'Go away, you're in great health,' but only until the symptoms materialise again; and then often they seem much worse. If no one believes your symptoms are real, does it mean it's all in your mind? Or, worse still, incurable?

People who already have asthma, heart disease or chronic pain symptoms may be made worse by erratic over-breathing. Often, instead of recognising hyperventilation, their doctors load them with extra drugs for the existing condition. This is hardly surprising since medical training has in recent years offered only passing mention of the subject of hyperventilation – usually just the acute phase. This results in a focus only on symptoms.

Doctors often treat the individual symptoms of HVS, not the underlying disorder causing all the distress. It's rather like prescribing skin lotion to someone with yellow jaundice.

Where to start?

One doctor described hyperventilation syndrome as 'a diagnosis begging for recognition'. Once it has been diagnosed, though, there are a number of possible treatments that your doctor may offer.

Drug options

The most common drugs prescribed are tranquillisers, which may be life-savers in the short term but leave the habitual over-breathing component untreated. Long-term use of these exposes you to the added risks of dependency and addiction – and a greater loss of self-reliance.

Courses of antidepressants which are physically

non-addictive are worth considering when disabling anxiety, fearfulness or phobias exist. They can be seen as a 'chemical holiday', rebuilding levels of serotonin (a mood enhancer) worn down by stress. They can provide shelter from the storm: room to restore normal breathing patterns and develop an effective relaxation response.

Physical coping skills

Long-term 'bad breathers' benefit from physiotherapy sessions both for breathing retraining and for sorting out the complex physical side-effects that radiate from HVS and its symptoms. Musculo-skeletal problems commonly add to the mix and need special attention.

Upper-chest breathing requires sustained effort from accessory muscles, which were primarily designed for a supporting role only. Physical symptoms such as headaches, costochondritis (painful rib joints), neck and shoulder stiffness and pain result, and add to the general misery. Physical changes literally 'fix' the upper chest muscles.

Mental coping skills

Some chronic hyperventilators develop avoidance behaviours in an attempt to control symptoms by controlling their environment. Perpetual anxiety about maintaining control is a common cause of phobias. The most common of these are:

- fear of being away from home (agoraphobia)
- fear of enclosed spaces (claustrophobia)
- fear of travel, either driving or flying.

Anxiety about sex may also lead to avoidance

through fear of symptoms, fear of failure, or fear of not being able to cope with intense emotion.

Expert psychiatric or psychological help would be advisable if these problems continued.

The BETTER Breathing Plan

The options listed above do not provide the whole answer, although they are a valid and vital part of treatment.

There is another treatment, one that is simple, although it requires like most things commitment to change. The six-step plan detailed in the next section uses the letters BETTER to cover important aspects of recovery.

> **B** Breathing retraining
> **E** Esteem
> **T** Total body relaxation
> **T** Talk
> **E** Exercise
> **R** Rest and sleep

Read on and discover how to combat HVS and restore normal breathing (and blood gases) and look at ways to cope with the pressures causing these problems. Use the charts at the back to monitor your progress. And 'when in doubt, breathe out'.

'This breathing business is to do with shedding some of the clutter that constricts us as tightly as our grandmothers' corsets. It's about embracing a sense of something special, easily and immediately accessible right there inside us, like an echo from childhood . . .'
Pru, 55

PART 2

The
BETTER
Breathing Plan

The BETTER Breathing Plan: B

Breathing Retraining
'The most crucial step was to start a daily practice.
No big deal – just five minutes of breathing down
into my belly, concentrating on the exhale,
embracing the stillness before the inhale. It was
ridiculously hard at first. Then it became as
effortless and essential as a morning pee. Five
minutes soon slipped into 10 then 20 minutes.'

Jenny 54

For people with chronic hyperventilation and
disordered breathing patterns, restoring a normal
breathing pattern takes a great deal of patience and
concentration, as well as regular practice. Some are
able to switch easily back to normal breathing,
while others may take months, sometimes up to a
year to be free of symptoms. It may be
uncomfortable at first, but using conscious effort to
restore your natural unconscious pattern enables
the respiratory control centres in your brain to reset
from overdrive back to normal.

The following simple techniques will help turn
you into a good breather, although you may need

extra help. A session with a respiratory physiotherapist is a good way to check out any musculo-skeletal or postural problems that may have developed, and to cover coping strategies for stress and tension. It's much easier to learn from a hands-on assessment.

The four basic steps in breathing retraining are:

- becoming aware of faulty breathing patterns
- learning low, slow nose-breathing
- learning to relax the upper chest and shoulders
- restoring normal breathing volumes and rates (10–14 breaths per minute).

Big versus deep breaths

From a very early age, often at school, people learn to stick out their chests and suck in their stomachs like soldiers or *Baywatch* stars. Ask anyone to take a deep breath and chances are they'll fill up their whole chest and take a *big* breath instead.

Try it. Stand in front of a mirror and place the hand you write with on your stomach between your lower ribs and navel. Then put the other hand on your breast-bone, just below your collarbone.

Take a deep breath and observe three things.

- Which part of your chest moved first?
- Which part of your chest moved most?
- Did you breathe in through your nose or mouth?

If you breathed in through your nose, your stomach expanded first and you felt minimal upper chest movement, you executed a true deep breath, reflecting a natural breathing pattern.

If you breathed in fast through your mouth, and

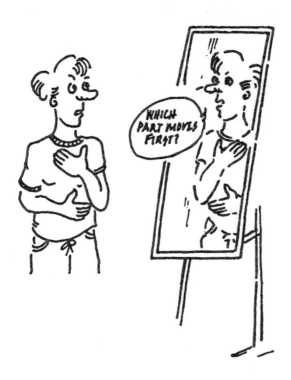

you could see and feel your upper chest heave first, and you felt little or no stomach movement or drew it *in,* you might have a disordered breathing pattern.

Strategies for breathing retraining

It's best to start out by practising lying comfortably on your back. This means you can switch off all your postural reflexes and relax your whole body while you retrain. Most people agree it's easier to focus on abdominal breathing this way while relearning the natural pattern. Getting the knack of abdominal breathing lying down makes the progression to it while sitting and standing easier.

Lying with a pillow under your head and knees, concentrate on the out breath. You may find it easier at first to lie with your hands clasped behind your head, to relax the upper chest muscles. Let the air 'fall' out of your chest without pushing. Breathe in gently through your nose and let go straight away, concentrating on breathing out lightly. Shoulder and upper chest relaxation is vital.

With lips together and jaw loose, draw air lightly in through your nose, relaxing and expanding your waist, feeling your stomach puff up. Let go straight away and allow the elastic recoil of your diaphragm and lower chest to breathe air out effortlessly and quietly.

If you feel dizzy it means you're still big-breathing rather than deep-breathing. Cup both hands over your mouth and nose and rebreathe carbon dioxide-rich air for five or six breaths, then rest. Repeat this until the dizzies have gone.

Start with very light, small abdominal breaths. Make sure you let go straight away at the top of the in-breath – don't hold – and that you relax at the end of the breath out. If you feel like taking huge draughts of air in, resist the temptation. Remember: if you breathe in big you're going to breathe out big too, further depleting carbon dioxide levels.

Silently repeat to yourself, 'Lips together, jaw relaxed, breathing low and slow.' This mental chant helps concentration.

Imagine a piece of fine elastic around your waist stretching as you inhale. Or think of breathing into

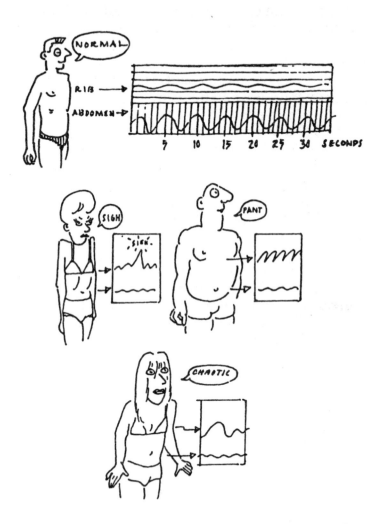

your (loose) belt or waistband. Check chest movements with your hands.

Spend at least 10 minutes per session. Repetition is essential.

Timing

Once you feel confident about your breathing pattern, concentrate on the rate.

Time yourself by watching the seconds hand on a watch or clock for half a minute while you count your breaths (breathing in and out is one breath). Aim to breathe at about 12 breaths a minute – six per half minute.

If you are much faster than that, relax, let go and check again in a couple of minutes. If you are too much slower, lighten your breathing – and relax.

The relaxed pause at the end of exhalation means breathing out takes longer than breathing in. One imaginative man found that it helped his timing to, instead of counting, mentally say the words 'Bombay' (breathe in) 'Sapphire' (breathe out) 'Gin' (relax)!

Exhalation may be more prolonged (Sapp-h-i-r-e) in people with chest disorders such as asthma, or chronic obstructive respiratory diseases. This is normal.

Keeping up the practice

Practise the new low, slow breathing pattern lying on your side, sitting and standing. When you walk or go up and down stairs, synchronise your breathing with movement. For example, breathe in for two steps, out for three.

At first, if you've been addicted to mouth/upper-chest breathing, nose/abdominal breathing will feel peculiar. Some describe it as 'back to front' breathing. Others report uncomfortable feelings of air hunger. This is a good sign showing you are making progress. Your respiratory centre is being challenged to accept normal carbon dioxide levels and will try and make you 'big-breathe' again.

When you feel breathless
STOP – check your chest
DROP – relax shoulders and upper chest
FLOP – relax all over
Use rest positions (see opposite) whenever and wherever you get short of breath.
Focus on low, slow nose-breathing.

It may take a long time and a great deal of practice to get your diaphragm strong and working confidently, and for your respiratory centre to accept normal blood gas levels again. Don't be hard on yourself if you slip back into erratic patterns. Just concentrate on the next breath and getting it right.

Set the alarm five minutes early and every morning, before you get out of bed, lie on your back for a few minutes practising low, slow relaxed breathing. Establish the pattern for the day.

For the first week of retraining schedule two 10-minute sessions in the lying down position each day, morning and evening. Reduce to once a day in week two. Step up to twice a day again after bad days or stressful times.

During the day, every hour on the hour, check your chest, correct your breathing and *forget it*. Regular repetition is the best way to reinforce healthy breathing patterns – but don't be obsessive.

In bed at night repeat the morning breathing

Rest positions

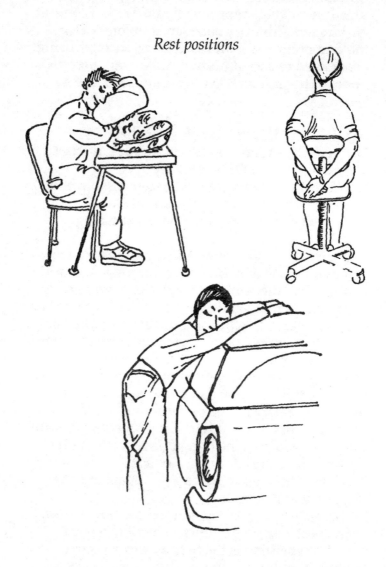

routine lying on your left side to help you go to sleep.

As you become re-accustomed to breathing properly, there will be less need to check the chest often. During stressful times, however, it pays to check breathing rates and patterns. Concentrating on this physical aspect helps dampen anxieties.

Common mistakes and problems

• Your diaphragm may be a bit jumpy at first, especially if it has been out of action for a while. Like any other group of muscles which have been out of use, your diaphragm may need strengthening.

If you find yourself breathing in a jerky 'staircase' fashion, mildly resisted breathing helps. A two-kilogram bag of rice placed just below the navel while lying down is ideal. (One woman found her iron made a perfect weight.) If you have problems with gastric reflux (heartburn), practise in a semi-reclining position.

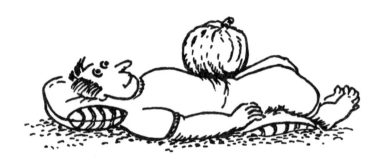

• Those on courses of steroid tablets, such as prednisone, need to pay special attention to maintaining diaphragm strength. Loss of condition in larger muscle groups, for example, thigh muscles, is a common side-effect and can weaken the diaphragm too. Strengthening exercises restore muscle power. Talk to your physiotherapist.

• Those with asthma – children and adults – need to pay special attention to their breathing after a bout of wheezing. Breathing may be chaotic during an attack, switching from upper to lower chest with little chance of control; this is normal – an increased respiratory drive is natural at this time.

Using rest positions and the 'stop, drop, flop' routine helps combat the stress and fear while waiting for the asthma medications to work. Once the attack is over, re-establishing low-volume nose-breathing and relaxing the upper chest must be top priority.

• Your body will play all sorts of tricks to start you over- breathing again. The urge to sigh, yawn or gulp air will seem overwhelming at times, and very uncomfortable at first. Remember this is a sign of progress: your respiratory centres are frantically trying to make you hyperventilate again. With regular and determined practice your respiratory centres will adjust to accept a balanced pH and normal ventilation.

To resist the urge to over-breathe, try swallowing hard and continue breathing low and slow.

• Wearing tight-fitting clothes and pulled-in belts restricts normal breathing. Loosen up. Wear braces or elasticised belts. During strong exercise, while it's normal to mouth-breathe to inhale extra oxygen, don't forget to resume nose-breathing as soon as you can after effort.

• Another popular mistake is to 'brace' or fill up the upper chest, holding in huge volumes of air while using the diaphragm to breathe in more. Breathing this way makes symptoms worse.

It is just as important to relax the upper chest and shoulders as it is to breathe low/slow/nose.

A relaxing image to use in focusing on low, slow nose-breathing is to imagine breathing in through your heels.

When you feel your breathing is high in your chest remember to:

• relax your shoulders by using a rest position (see page 70);
• keep lips together, jaw relaxed, shoulders dropped;
• concentrate on low, slow nose-breathing until you feel calm.

In other words, stop, drop, flop.

'I've changed my life by changing the way I breathe. It feels dramatic, a magical shift for me. Nothing looks different from the outside – it's just that every day I feel lighter, at ease.'

Jenny, 54

7

The BETTER Breathing Plan: E
Esteem

'Looking through some photos of about five or six years ago, I was struck by how confident and "together" I looked then. Remembering those times made me realise how down I was now, and how timid I'd become never sure if I was going to be OK or not in different situations. A recent photo showed me with my shoulders up to my ears nearly and looking pretty glum. I really had lost a lot of confidence in myself.'

Peter, 31

Most chronic hyperventilators suffer from a battered self-image. Good days may be few and far between, and these are overshadowed by the fear and loathing of bad days. Gradual erosion of confidence – feeling you are letting yourself or your friends down – adds to the general lack of self-worth. Strong positive emotions such as love, happiness and laughter gradually get pushed aside by anxiety, anger (often repressed) and depression.

While you might receive support during times of

major personal upheaval, little attention is paid to the cumulative effects of minor everyday niggles.

If left unresolved these can build up to major proportions. The skill of being able to say, 'Sorry, but no . . .' to demands you know will overload you is a very important one to master.

The power of laughter

Loosening up, relaxing and finding some humour in your life will prove that laughter is a powerful chemical-free remedy. Laughter benefits the whole person, body and soul; a good belly laugh liberates the mind from repetitive, often negative, thought patterns.

One group of researchers found increased levels of immunoglobulins (antibodies) were produced in people watching funny films over those watching dreary ones. Laughter also seems to reduce the output of the stress hormone adrenalin and, just as exercise releases opioid peptides (hormones that make you feel good), so does laughter. The final bonus is the exquisite relaxation that follows laughter and enjoyment.

Use of language

Breaking the *tension* $\Rightarrow$ *HVS* $\Rightarrow$ *anxiety* $\Rightarrow$ *HVS* cycle requires a firm commitment to a change in outlook as well as breathing patterns. Language and choice of words play an important role. To start with, cross the words 'should', 'if only' and 'what if' out of your vocabulary.

Being aware of negative or illogical thought and speech patterns helps you to change them. Listen to yourself. If you catch yourself thinking, 'I'll never be able to manage . . .' or 'I'm always letting people

down . . .', gently question yourself. Always?
Never? Think about it.

Depression

Fear of losing control is especially strong in chronic
hyperventilators. This often leads to repression of
normal emotions and the withholding of love,
warmth, anger or sadness. Unexpressed grief, fear
or resentment puts you in the fast lane to
depression and withdrawal from everyday knock-
about life.

At the risk of giving depression a good name, it is
a fairly normal reaction to prolonged bouts of
symptomatic hyperventilation. If there is nothing

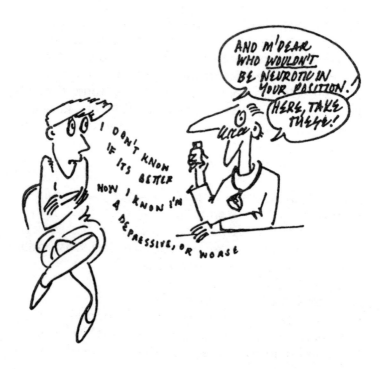

obvious to cut out or to take a pill for, anxiety and depression are reasonable enough reactions to feeling constantly off key. Treating the symptoms with drugs without paying attention to the breathing disorder is going to be of limited value to the sufferer, and of great expense to our already overstretched health-care system.

More sinister, though, with the accompanying wearing away of self-esteem comes the likelihood of turning hyperventilators into chronic invalids. If the patient is shunted from specialist to specialist trying to find a diagnosis, undergoing all sorts of invasive or risky investigations with no relief, it's not surprising anxiety and depression become chronic.

Stress

Stress is essential to life – we'd be dead without it. But too much can lead to us ending up dead too.

One thing we can consciously control when managing stress responses is our breathing, which has a direct and indirect effect on the way we react. On the other hand, once your nervous system starts signalling 'Stress attack!', abusing stimulants (coffee, cigarettes, alcohol or recreational drugs) to boost flagging energy levels is asking for trouble.

Good ways to prevent overreaction to stressors include:

• accepting that it's how we respond to stress, not the stress itself, that does the damage;
• realising that breathing in excess of metabolic need affects all our body systems;
• understanding that breathing, while mostly automatic, is also under conscious control;
• using breathing techniques to help us avoid body

chemistry imbalances and the symptoms caused by over-breathing.

Restoring a strong and healthy self-image means you're more likely to take notice of your body's reactions to stress, tiredness and the early signs of exhaustion.

Think about lifestyle changes to reduce stress levels. Schedule time for breathing retraining, relaxation, massage, exercise and sleep to absorb the effects of stress.

Body mechanics and posture

Good posture is a very important ingredient in combating HVS.

Check regularly: imagine being suspended by a fine thread from the back of the top of your head.

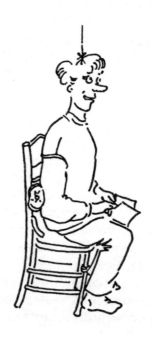

Stretch up tall to prevent breaking this phantom thread.

Always sit with your bottom snug against the back of the chair. Maintaining a lumbar hollow in sitting stops your upper spine sagging and compressing your lower chest and gut. Apart from the mechanical advantages to the process of breathing itself, holding and carrying yourself well – standing or sitting – is a good look, helping restore physical confidence.

Tell a friend

A potent way of taking the fear out of HVS is to tell *five* people you know about it. Explain the symptoms, how they start and how you handle them. You'll be surprised how many other people have experienced it.

Unravelling the tight spiral of HVS can be a long yet illuminating process. Gaining insight into the mechanisms that bring on HVS is only the starting point though. Dealing with its effects may need extra assistance. Plenty of help exists out in the community to help rebuild a healthy self-image if you need it.

Family, individual and group counselling is available from a variety of agencies. Check out your local library for information. Browse through the dozens of excellent self-health books on the shelves.

Coming to grips with HVS, and getting it off your chest, will put you back in the driving seat and in, not under or out of, control.

'When it was pointed out to me, I saw it was so true. I used negative language against myself

nearly all the time. On top of that I seemed to sigh every time I finished saying anything. Especially after being on the phone. It was such a habit!'

Rose, 41

8

The BETTER Breathing Plan: T
Total Body Relaxation

'I felt very restless and uncomfortable even thinking about my breathing. When I lay on my back I felt incredibly tense. I was asked to clasp my hands behind my head. It was amazing because immediately I could feel my lower chest and diaphragm area working properly without even trying. Soon I felt intensely relaxed – I actually started to laugh, I felt so bloody good. It wasn't nervous laughter – just a fantastic letting go.'

Peter, 31

If you've been struggling for weeks, months or even years with chronic hyperventilation, bizarre symptoms, fear and tension, you may find it extremely hard to let go and relax. Releasing physical tension helps release mental tension – the rats-in-the-brain repetitive thoughts that spin through your mind – but this negative internal chatter-box may be just as hard to subdue as trigger-happy lungs.

Learning the knack of switching on relaxation when familiar hyperventilation symptoms reappear – and they will in times of stress – is an effective way of stopping symptoms in their tracks. It's difficult at first to feel you can release tension or to feel you can take time out to practise relaxation techniques. But daily dips into the relaxation response pay off, giving you more reserves to cope with the daily pressures – good and bad – which are part of normal life.

Remember that all relaxation methods start with low, slow nose-breathing, so mastering chapter 6 is essential before continuing further.

Choosing a suitable relaxation method

There are plenty of methods to choose from. Your choice will depend on whether mental or physical tension is more of a problem, and where you are at the time. Knowing a variety of methods helps you be more adaptable.

Most public hospital physiotherapy out-patient departments teach various types of relaxation as part of general stress management. Check with your local hospital if you still have one.

The hyperventilator's special

The prone lying relaxation is ideal for hyper-ventilators. This involves lying on your front and especially suits people who feel vulnerable or ill-at-ease lying on their backs. Lying face down has a built-in sense of safety, with your soft underbelly protected by your spine.

The main elements of relaxation can be practised. These include:

- abdominal breathing
- switching off anti-gravity or postural reflexes
- arousing awareness of tension zones
- reducing sympathetic system tone (your body's stress response).

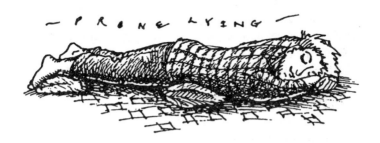

Preparation

Schedule a time – at least 10–15 minutes at first. Mark time out for relaxation breaks in your diary or daily chores list.

Choose a quiet place to practise and take the phone off the hook, or turn down the ring volume. Tell those around you what you are doing and why, and ask not to be disturbed. Even quite young children can be co-operative about 'your time' and may even enjoy time-keeping.

Technique

Lying face down on a bed, put a firm pillow under your hips to free the diaphragm, and under your ankles to relax your back. You may need a soft pillow under your upper chest if you have a stiff neck.

If you can lie with your arms up, hands under your brow, this helps suppress upper-chest breathing, as in the forward-leaning rest position (see page 70). If your shoulders are uncomfortable, keep your arms by your sides.

Don't go to sleep in this position if you have restricted neck movement.

You can practise some of the mental relaxation techniques (see below) or listen to soothing music. After initial concentration on breathing low and slow for three or four breaths, forget about breathing and . . . let go.

Relaxing this way is surprisingly rejuvenating.

Progressive muscle relaxation

This involves methodically stretching muscle groups for five or six seconds, and letting go for 10–15 seconds, concentrating on the difference between tension and release. It is an excellent way of pinpointing tension zones, such as your neck, scalp, shoulders, hands and lower back. Most people doing this relaxation technique for the first time are surprised at the amount of physical strain they've been holding on to, and even more surprised at how good it feels to let it go.

The whole process takes 10–15 minutes at first. But if you practise regularly you'll find it takes less and less time to switch off, and you can continue with 'mini-relaxes'. This technique is easy to learn and can be adapted to do while sitting in a chair, at work, or on planes, buses or trains.

Technique

1 Lie on your back, put a pillow under your head and knees, and cover up with a rug. Begin with two or three slow, light abdominal breaths, then forget your breathing.

2 Starting with your left leg, pull your toes up towards you, pressing the back of your knee into the pillow, tightening your whole leg to the hip (your heel will lift). Hold for five seconds – and let go slowly, relaxing for 10–15 seconds. Repeat with the right leg.

3 Continue with the same timing as you stretch and elongate the fingers and thumb of your left hand. Let go slowly . . . relax. Repeat with the right hand.

4 Push your left elbow gently into the bed. Let go slowly . . . relax. Repeat with the right elbow.

5 Slide your hands down the bed towards your feet, feeling the stretch to your shoulders and neck. Let go slowly . . . relax.

6 Tuck in your chin and gently press your head back into the pillow, stretching the long muscles up the back of your neck. Let go slowly . . . relax.

7 Very lightly bring your teeth together. With lips closed, separate your teeth a little and move your jaw slightly from side to side. Stop. Swallow hard and . . . relax, with the tip of your tongue behind your top front teeth.

8 Screw up your nose. Let go . . . relax.

9 Think of your eyelids as being light as feathers resting softly over your eyes. With eyes remaining closed, raise your eyebrows as high as you can . . . and let go slowly, feeling your brow and scalp smooth and relaxed. This is a common area of tension. Repeat two or three times.

10 Check tension zones and repeat sequences in those areas that still feel tight. At first you may have to repeat tensing/relaxing routines 10 or more times before you feel release.

11 When you feel you have unwound, rest and enjoy the feeling. Keep nagging or disruptive thoughts at bay by focusing on neutral repetitive ones, for example, mentally chanting your two times table.

Mental relaxation methods

There are many of these, but I will give details here only of the easiest. Look in your local library for relevant books and tapes. Make relaxation as important and regular as cleaning your teeth.

Passive mental relaxation

This involves sitting comfortably, eyes closed, hands on thighs, palms turned up.

Start with abdominal breathing. After three or four breaths, stop concentrating on breathing or trying to relax, but passively accept whatever floats through the mind. Focus your concentration by silent repetition of a short word (try repeating the word 'one' with each breath out).

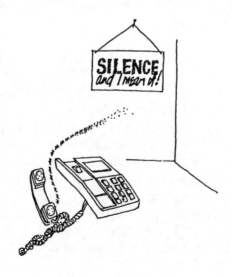

Along with mental relaxation, you will experience deep physical relaxation.

Transcendental meditation

Introduced to the West over 30 years ago, transcendental meditation (TM) is still a popular relaxation and meditation method. It's a type of passive mental relaxation, where an individual word is given, to be rapidly and silently repeated while focusing on deep physical and mental relaxation for 20 minutes twice a day. Nagging conscious thoughts are pushed out by the silent repetition of your given word.

Most major towns have a TM centre. It is relatively expensive, but for people who have difficulty getting started with relaxation the group support is helpful.

Auto hypnosis

This method involves sitting fully supported in a chair about three metres from a wall, focusing on a spot just above eye level.

Counting breaths back from 100, picture yourself floating and free. As your eyes start to feel heavy, let them close, and stop counting when you feel floppy and pleasantly relaxed. You will be fully awake and aware of your surroundings, and as soon as you want to finish, count three breaths to slowly revert to alert.

Creative visualisation

Creative visualisation involves relaxing around positive pleasurable mental images and has been shown to be intensely relaxing. By involving your senses – imagining tastes, smell, textures and sounds – you build up a rich picture in your mind.

About two billion brain cells make up our speech and thought centres. But our unconscious is made up of 100 billion brain cells, and our visual sense operates mainly in this larger area. No one has worked out why, but our brains don't differentiate between vividly imagined events and real ones. When you think about a painful or frightening situation your body reacts as though it is really happening, as in the think test (see page 56).

Recent experiments on the muscles of people with back pain showed that muscle tension increased between two and six times when the person being tested simply *thought* about their pain. Reversing this response makes sense. Relaxation with visualisations make a very potent natural relaxant.

To do creative visualisation, set yourself up as for other methods: sitting, or lying on your front or back. Remember, perhaps, a childhood picnic, reliving the sounds of the sea, sun on your skin, sand between your toes, the smell and textures of peeling an orange and its sweet taste.

Other ways of relaxing

• Yoga classes are an excellent way of combining exercise, breathing and relaxation. Most classes finish with a 20-minute total body relaxation. Joining a class is a good way for busy people to schedule time out without guilt. Shop around to find a class that suits you.

Avoid the more advanced breathing exercises at first. Stick to low volume abdominal breathing and explain why to your teacher if asked.

• Treating yourself to regular back or full body

massages from a reputable massage therapist is an excellent alternative to the more cerebral approaches to relaxation. Long-term hyperventilators often have stiff, tense upper spines with painful knotty muscles. Having these gently kneaded back into shape can make you feel you've had three relaxation sessions and a good night's sleep all rolled into one.

• Routinely practising gentle stretches of tense muscle groups is strongly recommended, especially if you have a sedentary job.

• Both men and women report the value of having a facial, which includes neck and upper chest massage. It is also another good way of scheduling time out.

• Dubbed by one wit as a 'wooden Valium', resting in a rocking chair is an excellent quick-fix relaxation method.

How often? How long?

Feeling good enough about yourself to take the time for yourself to relax is vitally important, and regular practice is a priority in recovery from HVS. The ideal is to weave two 10-minute sessions into your day. Experiment with different methods for different times of the day and week.

You may not feel much immediate benefit, and often it's other people who first remark on changes. It is essential to stick at it. Sometimes at the beginning unpleasant reactions to 'letting go' put hyperventilators off continuing with regular practice, but it is worth persevering, so try another method.

Regular practice increases your general awareness of stresses and strains and the need to let go shoulder and upper chest muscles. Once you develop an effective relaxation response, 'mini-relaxes' practised several times throughout the day are often sufficient – checking and releasing tension zones as you chest-check your breathing patterns. During the course of the day, check your shoulders, elbows and hands when walking, making sure they're loose and relaxed.

Just as you recognise triggers that bring on over-breathing, create some relaxation triggers of your own to combat it. Try mentally repeating, 'Lips together, jaw relaxed, breathing low and slow,' as you turn your palms up and drop your shoulders. Remind yourself how much energy you're wasting by being physically tense, and how continued tension undermines your sense of well being.

Remember – *relaxation only helps eliminate the symptoms, not the causes of stress.* It's important to develop 'the serenity to accept the things you cannot change, the courage to change the things you can, and the wisdom to know the difference' – to paraphrase the Alcoholics Anonymous dictum.

Addiction to bad breathing can be a hard habit to break.

'I must admit I thought "relaxation" was a bit too nerdy and navel-gazing for me. But when I learnt more about the relaxation response and how to switch it on at will without having to lie round going "om" for hours I was hooked. Short 'mini-relaxes' suit my busy lifestyle (which I enjoy) and prevent me lapsing back into my speedy hyper ways.'

Barbara, 30

9

The BETTER Breathing Plan: T
Talk

'Whenever he thought he was about to speak in the tutorial, his breathing lost its regular pattern and he knew it was all over until he could regain control, which would allow his words to come out evenly and without the rushed delivery which made him sound as if he were speaking after a short uphill sprint . . .'

From The Miserables, *by Damien Wilkins*

Co-ordinating talking and breathing is often a major problem for over-breathers. There are two main reasons for this. The first is breath control is more difficult while speaking, and the second is that talking about the symptoms and the anxieties associated with HVS often triggers over-breathing.

Breath control while speaking

It's important to express ideas and emotions through the power of speech. But the use of quick, gasping upper-chest breaths while talking prompts HVS symptoms.

Slightly husky light speech, punctuated by throat clearing, sniffing, or yawning, often indicates hyperventilation. Marilyn Monroe's sexy, breathless voice may have had more to do with an overactive upper chest, her waist constricted by a cinch belt restricting normal low-chest breathing. A full-toned, confident voice needs good breath control: ask a barrister, actor or singer.

Try these techniques to improve breath control while speaking. If you continue to have a problem, get expert advice from a speech therapist. These tips also apply to people who have problems maintaining good breathing while eating.

• Relax both shoulders, and abdominal nose-breathe before speech.
• Draw air in through your nose between sentences while talking, instead of quickly upper-chest gasping through your mouth.
• Put mental commas and pauses into your speech.
• Practise speaking in front of a mirror. Recite the alphabet slowly. Chest-check to observe and correct chest movements.
• Practise reading aloud from a book and tape record yourself. It's interesting to monitor progress by repeating this every couple of weeks.
• Watch other people's breathing patterns when they speak, and listen during telephone conversations. See if you can pick another bad breather.
• Be aware of centring your breathing – low and slow.
• Combining eating and talking with breathing is a challenge for some. Most of the best advice about relaxed eating was given to us by our parents. Sit

down to eat – and avoid eating on the run or talking with your mouth full. This is a fast track to air-gulping and dyspepsia. Eat very small mouthfuls if 'tight throat' symptoms and fear of choking is a problem. Drink small sips to prevent air-gulping. Drinking through a straw is a good way to practise sipping and swallowing. Never eat while slumped in a low chair: avoid pressure from the stomach restricting diaphragm movement.

Repression and depression

Talking may be particularly difficult when you are voicing deep anxieties about HVS symptoms.

Bottling up problems is not good for your health. Anxiety increases mental and physical tension and accelerates adrenalin output. This revs up heart and breathing rates – and HVS symptoms. Recent scientific research has proved that thinking or talking about physical symptoms can both directly and indirectly affect your body chemistry.

The indirect physiological effect lies in the relationship between stress and the onset of exhaustion and depression. Losing control over parts of your life (as felt with chronic hyperventilation) is a major ingredient in some sorts of depression. A sense of isolation develops if you are afraid of confiding in anyone. It is worse still if you do and are thought neurotic.

Lacking confidence to handle social occasions or keep up friendships – or thinking you are letting family, friends or work mates down – is a common sign of anxiety and a potent depressant.

Can you hear me?

Listening skills often need brushing up as much as

talking skills: expression and communication are very much two-way processes. People close to you may have become alarmed, confused or even bored by your symptoms.

Relaxing enough to listen to other people is as necessary as finding someone who will listen to you.

Deciding to change

Scientific medicine, with high-tech surgical and pharmaceutical interventions, has revolutionised the healing arts over the last 30 years. But it has also produced an unrealistic belief in a 'magic bullet' as the cure-all, encouraging a passive attitude to becoming well. Recovery from hyperventilation requires active involvement and personal

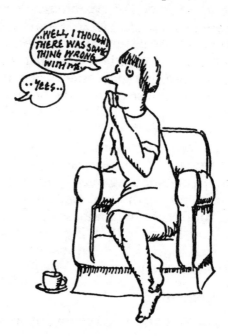

commitment. And talking – being able to identify triggers and confront the need for acceptance or change is a vital part of reducing the stress.

For those who have difficulty identifying the sources of their anxieties, sessions with a clinical psychologist, psychiatrist or psychotherapist can be of enormous benefit in speeding up recovery.

A resonant, confident voice comes with low, slow breathing, relaxation and talking out – releasing negative emotions. Find someone you trust to confide in. Use positive language. Starting with the next breath, talk yourself up and away from HVS symptoms.

'Reading stories to my children is a pleasure now. It used to be a nightmare. I used to read in a monotone without a break, then gasp in a lungful of air and try to carry on. Then I'd start to feel light-headed. The poor kids – it can't have been much fun for them. We all enjoy it now that I'm breathing properly.'

Elsa, 29

The BETTER Breathing Plan: E
Exercise

'When I got back into regular enjoyable exercise, I experienced a conceptual shift in that things that had stressed me out before no longer bothered me. I realised, too, that my inactivity had in itself been a stress.'

Max, 48

Breathing pattern disorders and low physical fitness levels tend to go hand in hand. This may be due to:

• fear of triggering uncontrollable rapid breathing during effort
• panic about not being able to breathe in enough air
• side-effects of poor sleep and exhaustion
• fear of fatigue.

Nearly all chronic hyperventilators complain of muscle fatigue. The most common types they mention are: central fatigue, with general feelings of low energy, and peripheral fatigue felt in limbs, where muscles tire quickly and ache from lactic acid build-up resulting from low carbon dioxide levels.

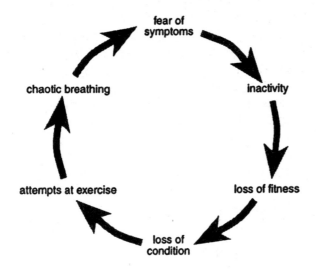

Why is physical fitness important in HVS?

The effects of inactivity – sluggish circulation, achy muscles, lack of energy and shortness of breath – not only make you feel below par but add to a general loss of self-confidence.

Fitness is defined as 'the body's ability to meet the normal demands of everyday life – work and recreation – with ease, and with enough margin to adequately cope with emergencies'. Most hyperventilators would admit falling far behind this description.

Everybody feels better when they have energy to spare. Being fit has added bonuses: it leads to improvement of body image and a stronger sense of self-reliance. Enjoyment of regular physical exercise and the sense of confidence it brings is a vital part of recovery from HVS.

Recent fitness recommendations have changed emphasis from an exercise training/fitness to a physical activity/health model 'which uniquely incorporates *moderate* intensity and *intermittent* physical activity'. This is good news for those who have become drastically inactive or who work long hours in sedentary jobs. It means you can divide up daily physical exercise into short episodes. For example, a brisk short walk in the morning, before lunch and after work.

As long as the accumulated time *gradually* increases towards a total of 30 minutes of brisk activity per day, six to seven days a week, it will provide basic health benefits. For most this is extremely easy to manage.

Getting started

Check with your doctor before starting a new activity programme.

Start building basic fitness with low impact exercise options. These include brisk walking, exercycling, low-resistance circuit training at a gym and swimming. Gardening, raking leaves, mowing lawns, playing outdoor games with your kids, going dancing and walking the dog are all excellent 'body boosters'.

A graduated walking programme is a safe, enjoyable and easy way to improve basic fitness. It's cheap and interesting (looking at your surroundings), and needs no special clothing except for comfortable walking shoes. A big advantage is being able to nose-breathe while exercising. Include a friend or partner who knows about your symptoms to 'fitten up' with you.

(If you don't like outdoor exercise, hire or buy an exercycle and increase cycling times as you would with walking.)

• Set yourself a time, not a distance, to walk (or exercycle). Decide for yourself, based on your symptoms, and err on the light side at first. You can start as low as three minutes.
• Increase by a minute a day or as symptoms allow. Do two or three sessions a day until your total exercising time reaches 30 minutes. Hyperventilators tend to be over-achievers: make sure progress is gradual. You can then choose whether to exercise once a day for 30 minutes, or have two 15-minute or three 10-minute sessions a day.
• At first limit yourself to walking on the flat. Make sure your shoulders and arms are loose and relaxed. Use a good arm swing and walk at a brisk pace. As you start to feel fitter and more confident, include slopes and hills. It's normal to puff going up hills – you need more oxygen. Take smaller strides and slow down. Stop and rest if you feel uncomfortable.
• If you start to feel breathless or experience chest symptoms, 'stop, drop, flop' immediately. Take up a rest position (see page 70). Chest-check and low, slow nose-breathe back to normal before continuing.
• Be prepared for ups and downs – some days will be harder than others. Gradually, though, your exercise tolerance and confidence will improve.

When you reach a level where you manage 30 minutes of brisk exercise a day with little or no symptoms or breathing problems, you have reached *a basic* level of fitness. This will be maintained if you exercise at the same level six or seven days a week.

The joys of walking include:

- aerobic benefits (heart/lung efficiency)
- improved digestion and bowel function
- improved sleeping patterns
- relaxation.

For variety, include other ways of exercising.

- Use the stairs at work. Walk up one flight, or down two, before taking the lift.
- Try a rebounder, bouncing to your favourite music.
- Yoga and t'ai chi classes are especially recommended, combining breathing, exercise (especially flexibility) and relaxation.
- Whacking games – tennis, badminton and squash – are great for people needing to release anger, resentment or frustration.
- Join a dance class.
- Go swimming or aqua-jogging. You may need extra help with breathing co-ordination – check with the instructor.

Eating and exercise

Good nutrition is an important aspect of fitness, and many authorities cite bad diet as a major source of stress. Not eating properly and not getting enough exercise often go together, and lead to physical neglect. This drastically increases the potential for sickness and misery.

If you are overweight, regular exercise helps weight loss. You feel less like eating directly after exercise, so if you are trying to lose weight, exercising shortly before meals helps tone down the appetite.

If you are underweight, take care to avoid heavy endurance types of exercise and concentrate on flexibility and low-resistance activities well before meals.

Skipping meals and relying on junk foods to boost flagging energy levels will only add to an already overburdened nervous and metabolic system.

Hyperventilators tend to interpret their fatigue as being due to low blood sugar (hypoglycaemia). But sugar is not, and never has been, an essential part of our diet. The sugar 'high' after eating sweets is short-lived. The body's production of the hormone insulin soon clears the high blood-sugar level and works to restore a normal balance, resulting in a slump in energy. Reaching for more high-sugar food only continues the cycle. Choose protein snacks instead (nuts or cheese) as these keep blood-sugar levels steadier longer. For this reason, a high-protein diet is recommended if you are prone to panic attacks. Experiment and see for yourself.

Alcohol, another high sugar source, tends to also accelerate the heart rate, fuelling over-breathing. While one beer or a glass of wine is an excellent relaxant, more may be asking for trouble.

Smoking

Smoking is another habit that complicates an over-breather's life. It's not hard to imagine the chaos that strong inhalations of smoke wreak upon your already hyper-breathing and overworked upper chest muscles.

Try to give up smoking while you are retraining your breathing. Join a smoking cessation group. See if you can spot fellow over-breathers.

It's usually more difficult giving up the rituals of smoking, and for hyperventilators that includes that first tidal inhalation after lighting up. Every time you think of the pleasures of smoking, give equal time to acknowledging the harmful effects and what it's doing to your heart and breathing rates. Consider whether you use smoking as an opportunity to hyperventilate. Dope smokers are especially prone to do this.

Think about what sort of smoker you are.

- If you smoke to relax, try a 'mini-relax' instead.
- If you smoke to give yourself a lift – go for a stroll in the fresh air or do some stretches instead.
- If you smoke because of the ritual of handling cigarettes and other smoking devices, invest in some worry beads to occupy your hands.

Remember: smoking heavily is asking for trouble. Stopping is best, cutting down helps.

Active again

Regular enjoyable exercise helps release naturally occurring opioid peptides into the bloodstream, and these make you feel good. Bones are kept strong too, which is especially important for those on courses of steroids and for post-menopausal women.

Movement, and pleasure in physical action, are basic human needs. Regular enjoyable activity is very much part of recovery from HVS.

'**The combination of loss of fitness and fear of symptoms made me dread the thought of exercise. I used to love running, but after a couple of frightening experiences of shortness of breath I thought I must have something wrong with my heart. But my heart was fine. My breathing wasn't though. The cardiologist I saw pointed out my disordered breathing and referred me for physiotherapy. I've gradually restored fitness, and enjoy running again.'**

Ted, 47

The BETTER Breathing Plan: R
Rest and Sleep

'Sleep *noun* the condition or period during which the mind and body rest, and voluntary movements and full consciousness are suspended.'

From the *Heinemann New Zealand Dictionary*

Rest and refreshing sleep are essential to good health: sound sleep provides a total release from the pressures of daily life. Very few people get through life, however, without from time to time experiencing muddled sleep patterns from extremes of either happiness or sadness. Someone newly in love seems hardly to need to sleep at all, and feels no worse for it. But most people find that during periods of stress or sickness the body demands more sleep.

Erratic sleep and vivid or bad dreams are very common hyperventilation syndrome symptoms, and being deprived of satisfying sleep causes a great deal of distress to an already overstretched nervous system. Worry about symptoms of HVS may be one reason for sleeplessness. But when

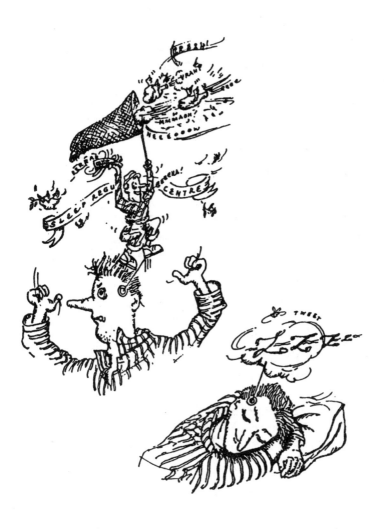

dreams and nightmares wake you with a pounding heart and in a panic, sleep itself may become feared.

Normal sleep

Sleep is controlled from a regulating centre deep in the brain stem. It processes information from all parts of the body joints, muscles, organs – as well as from the higher thought centres of the brain, or cerebral cortex. A low level of stimulation induces sleep, while a high level of stimulation leads to wakefulness. A calm mind as well as a calm body is necessary for satisfying sleep.

Sleep goes in cycles. The first main cycle is quiet sleep, which is true rest, with a *quiet* brain. It lasts about an hour. This is followed by rapid eye movement (REM) sleep, a shorter cycle of roughly 20–30 minutes. This is dream time and the brain is *active*.

During quiet sleep the body's metabolic rate, blood pressure and heart rate lower slightly and breathing is deep and regular. In REM sleep the heart beats up to 5 per cent faster, there is a slight increase in blood pressure and metabolic rate, the eyes dart about under closed lids – and breathing becomes irregular.

The average sleep needed for an adult is seven-and-a-half hours – five complete cycles. Individual patterns vary widely according to age, health and personality.

Why do people with HVS have sleep problems?

People with HVS are more sensitive to small fluctuations in carbon dioxide levels in their blood. The irregular breathing during REM sleep acts on the unconscious mind producing vivid or nightmarish dreams and lack of satisfying sleep. Another factor is the respiratory centre in the brain, which has become accustomed by day to lower carbon dioxide levels. By night it sends 'speed up' signals to the habitual hyperventilator – who may be sinking into relaxed deep breathing during quiet sleep. Feeling sensations similar to the air hunger felt at the start of breathing retraining, the sleeper wakes gasping for air.

Stress levels, high enough during waking hours, are raised further by disturbed rest and the exhaustion caused by poor sleep. Once natural breathing patterns are restored during the day natural sleep patterns return at night. For some this happens quickly, but for others it takes time and a great deal of patience and understanding to escape the downward spiral of wakefulness, worry, nightmares and sleeplessness.

Drugs and sleep

Short courses of antidepressants can be very helpful in restoring a normal sleeping pattern. They help replace chemicals and hormones depleted by

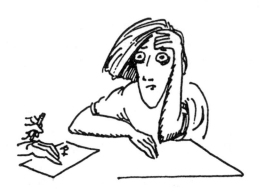

stress and lack of refreshing sleep. Some of these drugs are mild muscle relaxants too, which help reduce physical tension and chronic aches and pains. As they are not physically addictive, be open-minded if this option is suggested.

Sleeping pills are often a blessing for short stressful times, but if used for more than two weeks continuously they cease to work effectively and become addictive.

If you are dependent on sleeping pills, the information in this chapter will be of little use at first: withdrawal from sleeping pills must be gradual and with your doctor's help. Use the Good Sleep Plan once you have decided to make a success of getting off 'sleepers'.

The Good Sleep Plan

Try these simple strategies and give yourself time to re-establish a refreshing sleep pattern. Let your family and friends know your plans. If you share a bed, your partner will need to know.

Going to bed

• For the duration of retraining fix a regular time to go to bed and get up in the morning. Never go to bed earlier or get up later than these appointed times.
• Make your bedroom a stress-free zone. No TV, telephone, noisy clock, personal computer or radio.
• Small changes, such as new bed linen or moving the bed, can help start a new routine and break old associations.
• Soft, low lighting creates a restful atmosphere.

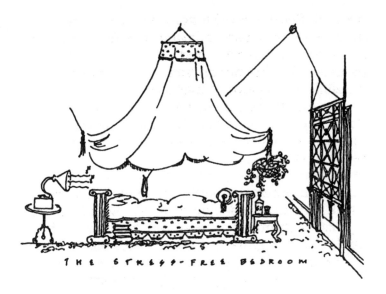

THE STRESS-FREE BEDROOM

- Use the bed for sleeping: no reading, sewing, eating, writing letters, talking on the phone.
- Making love is the only exception. Satisfying sex is a powerful prelude to relaxed sleep. Unfortunately, deep post-orgasmic relaxation lasts only four or five minutes, so if you haven't fallen asleep by then, it is of no added benefit. Seek expert help if anxiety about sex is a problem.
- Avoid rich, heavy or late-night dinners or Chinese food (high in monosodium glutamate) at the end of the day.
- Cut out coffee and strong tea for a month (try decaf). Gradually reintroduce it, and even then avoid it after 4 pm. If you're a heavy coffee drinker be ready for withdrawal symptoms – headaches, irritability and shakiness. Drink plenty of water.
- Avoid TV news and talkback radio for a month as well: watch light or funny programmes or videos

instead. Reduce extremes of positive (late-night movies) as well as negative (arguments) stimulation three or four hours before bed.

• Exercise helps reduce stress and induce sleep – if possible within four or five hours of bedtime.

• Have a warm, not hot, bath or shower before bed. Oil of lavender is an age-old remedy for relaxing mind and body. Add drops to the bath water or on the corner of your pillow.

• Cut out day sleeps. Daytime 'tiredness' is often the result of boredom or lack of activity. Go for a stroll instead of snoozing.

• Try warm milk as a night-cap. Milk has high levels of tryptophan, a naturally occurring enzyme which the body digests and converts into serotonin. This 'sleep nectar' has a powerful influence in promoting good moods and sound sleep.

(Tryptophan in tablet form has been available in New Zealand for over 30 years as a non-addictive 'natural' alternative to sleeping pills. Research in the US and Europe linked high dosages with a sometimes fatal blood disorder; contaminated stocks were thought to be responsible. As long as there is doubt about the tablets, rely on dietary intakes of tryptophan found in protein-rich foods such as milk, cheese, fish, meat and chicken.)

• Sedative herb teas such as passiflora and chamomile are safe alternatives for those who don't like milk.

• Write a list of things to be remembered or done the following day so you don't worry about tomorrow today. Constantly projecting into the future (or past) is a sure-fire sleep killer.

• Avoid going to bed on an unresolved fight or argument.

Getting off to sleep

Based on the sleep-retraining method devised by
US physician Richard Bootzin, the following regime
has proved extremely successful. Those who have
tried this scheme and stuck to it find it takes
between two and six weeks to start working and
say it is well worth the effort in restoring refreshing,
drug-free sleep. You can also try this approach if
you wake during the night.

• Once in bed and ready to sleep, lie on your back
and practise low, slow abdominal breathing
(through the nose) and relaxation techniques. Check
tension areas, stretch and release.
• Lie in a comfortable position (usually on the left
side to start) and glance at the time.
• If after 15 minutes you are still awake, get out of
bed. Go into another room and do something else
(read, watch a funny video, play patience, listen to
soothing music).
• When you feel ready for sleep, go back to bed
and if again you are not asleep within 15 minutes
repeat the sequence until you go to sleep.

**Learn to associate bed with sleep. If you're not
sleeping, don't stay in bed.**

Waking

• If your appointed waking time happens to come
in the middle of a deep, quiet sleep cycle you may
find it hard to wake. Don't interpret this as 'waking
up tired'. Many admit they let this feeling colour
their whole day, but all it means is you've woken

from a deep sleep cycle.
• If your appointed waking time comes towards the end of a REM sleep cycle, you'll wake up more alert, with fleeting memories of dreams.
• If nightmares wake you with hyperventilation symptoms, sit up and recover in a rest position (see page 70). Concentrate on relaxing your neck and shoulders and low, slow nose-breathing. When your breathing and heart rates have slowed, lie down to sleep again knowing over-breathing is the problem and you have techniques to combat it.

People who go to bed expecting not to sleep are often proved right. Breathing control and relaxation reduce tension and hyperventilation-induced symptoms. Your poor sleep pattern *can* be changed – and a refreshing one restored.

If you continue to have problems consult a sleep specialist.

'It was really strange going for a six-month check-up after my treatment for hyperventilation syndrome. Going over the list of symptoms I'd had at my first session, I couldn't believe it was me. But there it was, all written down. I'm so well now. My sleep patterns are normal, I no longer have those awful symptoms or fears about my health – I've forgotten all about them. It seems when you're unwell that's all you think about. I certainly appreciate feeling healthy again – but, strangely, I don't think about it.'

Trish, 36

Workbook

**Have your symptoms checked by your doctor
before starting breathing retraining. Check again
if symptoms continue to worry you.**

Commit to regular practice

Completing these charts is a graphic way of finding
how your stress levels, sleep and symptom patterns
interrelate with each other and with you.

Start with the 'Identification of Symptoms' chart.
This gives you a picture of how you are on day 1, at
the start of breathing retraining. At the beginning of
week 2, check symptoms on that day. Repeat on day
1 of week 3.

You can then compare progress from one week to
the next. Try not to look at the chart in between
times – paper clip the page to' the previous one.

Fill in the other charts daily for the next fortnight.
See if you can identify any patterns.

You should get an idea of what triggers to look
out for. Adapt your practice routines accordingly to
abolish symptoms.

Identification of symptoms

Listed here are some typical HVS symptoms. You
may have only a few of these symptoms while
others have the lot.

Start this chart the day you start breathing retraining. Compare day 1 (week 1) with day 1 (week 2) and then day 1 (week 3).

Symptoms	Example	Week 1	Week 2
Chest wall pains			
Physical tension	✓✓✓		
Tiredness	✓✓		
Visual disturbances			
Dizziness	✓		
Upset gut	✓		
Poor concentration	✓✓		
Faster or deeper breathing	✓✓✓		
Tight chest	✓✓		
Feeling revved up			
Tingling fingers			
Sighing/yawning	✓✓		
Tight jaw/throat	✓✓		
Headache			
Clammy/cold hands and feet	✓		
Erratic/faster heart beats	✓		
Others			

✓✓✓ = symptoms all day ✓✓ = some of the day ✓ = intermittent

Which situations trigger breathing discomfort?

Here are some situations that may trigger HVS.

Complete this chart, starting the day you begin breathing retraining, in the same way as the 'Identification of symptoms' chart. Compare day 1 (week 1) with day 1 (week 2) and then day I (week 3).

Triggers	Example	Week 1	Week 2
Driving			
Household chores			
Telephoning	✓✓		
High humidity			
Kissing/making love	✓		
Watching TV/cinema			
Talking	✓✓		
Meetings/interviews	✓✓✓		
Queues/crowds			
Exercise	✓✓		
Others			

✓✓✓ = always ✓✓ = often ✓ = sometimes

Stress and strain gauge

	Day 1			Day 2			Day 3			Day 4			Day 5			Day 6			Day 7		
	am	pm	n	am	pm	n	am	pm	n	am	pm	n	am	pm	n	am	pm	n	am	pm	n
10																					
9																					
8																					
7																					
6																					
5																					
4																					
3																					
2																					
1																					

	Day 8			Day 9			Day 10			Day 11			Day 12			Day 13			Day 14		
	am	pm	n	am	pm	n	am	pm	n	am	pm	n	am	pm	n	am	pm	n	am	pm	n
10																					
9																					
8																					
7																					
6																					
5																					
4																					
3																					
2																					
1																					

Every morning, afternoon and bedtime rate your
stress levels by putting a bold dot in the appropriate
box.

At the end of two weeks join the dots.

Compare this chart with your 'Symptoms',
'Eating' and 'Sleep' results (see opposite). Is there a
pattern?

1 = calm
10 = highly stressed
am = morning
pm = afternoon
 n = night

Symptoms
Breathing discomfort/sighing/air hunger

Day	1	2	3	4	5	6	7	8	9	10	11
Morning											
Afternoon											
Evening											
Night											

✓ = Yes, I am experiencing HVS symptoms.
O = I have no HVS symptoms.

Eating

Day	1	2	3	4	5	6	7	8	9	10	11
Breakfast											
Lunch											
Dinner											

✓ = Yes   ♥ = On the run   O = Skipped $ = Upset gut

Sleep

Day	1	2	3	4	5	6	7	8	9	10	11
No. of hours											
No. of wakes											
Wake refreshed? (✓ or O)											

Breathing retraining/'time out'/relaxing

Before you get out of bed, lie on your back and nose/abdominal breathe for a couple of minutes to establish your breathing pattern for the day.

In bed at night, low, slow nose-breathe while lying on your side to get off to sleep.

For the next two weeks, schedule time in the morning and afternoon or evening for 10 minutes' relaxed abdominal nose-breathing while lying. Make it a priority.

Day	1	2	3	4	5	6	7	8	9	10
Waking										
Morning										
Afternoon										
Night										

Be honest!

✓ = Yes   O = Forgot/no time

Conclusion

Breathing pattern disorders are alive and thriving in the 21st Century.

Definition and diagnosis have been contentious issues in recent years and continue to be the subject of lively international debate. However, enough 'sufferers' have responded to physiotherapy interventions involving breathing retraining, relaxation, postural adjustments and exercise prescriptions, and have enjoyed the far-reaching benefits of balanced blood gases, to make following the BETTER Breathing Plan a positive option.

Fifty per cent of the cure lies in knowing about and understanding the nature of hyperventilation syndrome. The rest is commitment to change.

Use the workbook again and again if you feel symptoms return during times of ill-health or stress. Reread the patients' stories and remember you are not alone.

Restoring normal low-chest breathing may take a long time. Don't be too hard on yourself if you do go off the rails and lapse back to disordered over-breathing.

Take a break. Take it seriously. Take the next energy efficient breath low and s l o w.

References

Chapter 1
L. C. Lum, 'Hyperventilation: The tip and the iceberg', *Journal of Psychosomatic Research*, vol. 19, 1976.
G. Magarian, 'Hyperventilation Syndrome: Infrequently recognised common expressions of anxiety and stress', *Medicine*, vol. 64 no. 4, 1982.
P. G. F. Nixon, 'Hyperventilation and Cardiac Symptoms', *Internal Medicine*, vol. 10 no. 12,1989.
J. Perera, 'The Hazards of Heavy Breathing', *New Scientist*, Dec. 1988.

Chapter 2
R. Freedman and S. Woodward, 'Behavioural Treatment of Menopausal Hot Flushes', *American Journal of Obstetrics and Gynecology*, 167, 1992.
Alexandra Hough, 'Physiotherapy for Survivors of Torture', *Physiotherapy*, vol. 78 no. 5, May 1992.
R.Schwarztstein et al., 'Dyspnoea: A sensory experience', *Lung*, 168, 1990.
John B. West, *Respiratory Physiology* (4th ed.), Williams and Wilkins, Baltimore, 1990.

Chapter 3
P. Chari, 'Acupuncture Therapy in Allergic Rhinitis', *American Journal of Acupuncture*, vol. 16 no. 2,1988.

R. Ley, 'Blood Breath and Fears: A hyperventilation theory of panic attacks and agoraphobia', *Clinical Psychology Review*, 8, 1988.
J. G. Widdicombe, 'The Physiology of the Nose', *Clinical Chest Medicine*, 7, 1986.
'The Work, Ways, Positions and Patterns of Nasal Breathing (relevance in heart and lung illness)', *Proceedings of the American Rhinologic Society*, 1972.

Chapter 4
W. N. Gardner, 'The Pathophysiology of Hyperventilation Disorders', *Chest*, 109, Feb.1996.
J. B. L. Howell, 'Behavioural Breathlessness', *Thorax*, 45, 1990.

Chapter 5
L. C. Lum, 'Psychogenic Breathlessness and Hyperventilation', Update May 1987.
B. Timmons and R. Ley (eds), Behavioural and Psychological Approaches to Breathing Disorders, *Plenum*, UK, 1994.

Chapter 6
Hough, 'Physiotherapy in Respiratory Care', 3rd edit., Nelson Thornes, 2001.
M. Thomas, R. K. McKinley, S. Mellor, G. Watkin, E. Holloway, J. Scullion et al. 'Breathing Exercises for Asthma: a randomized controlled trial', *Thorax*, 64, 2009.

Chapter 7
Susan Jeffers, *Feel the Fear and Do It Anyway*, Arrow, 2011.
Gail Ratcliffe, *Take Control of Your Life*, Doubleday New Zealand, 2011.

Chapter 8
Herbert Benson, *The Relaxation Response*,
Harper Collins, 2000.
Laura Mitchell, *Simple Relaxation*, John Murray,
1988.

Chapter 9
Donna Farhi, *The Breathing Book*, Simon and
Schuster, 1997.
Gwendoline Smith, *Sharing the Load*, Random
House, Auckland, 1996.

Chapter 10
Z. Altug and M. Miller, 'The Natural Exercise
Prescription', *Clinical Management*, vol. 9 no. 3.
Bob Anderson, Stretching, Shelter, 1997.
Wayne T. Phillips et al., 'Life Style Activity: Current
recommendations', *Patient Management*, November
1996.

Chapter 11
Fiona Johnston, *Getting a Good Night's Sleep*,
Random House New Zealand, 2005.

Index